High Speed Health

A Quick and Direct Guide to Healing Pain

Caused by Repetitive Strain Injuries

For the Part-Time Athlete

Who Sits at a Desk Full-Time

by Todd Bowen

www.highspeedhealth.com

The Sedentary Desk Jockey's Guide
to Health and Wellness Shortcuts

ISBN: 1500802182
ISBN 13: 9781500802189
Library of Congress Control Number: 2014914393
CreateSpace Independent Publishing Platform
North Charleston, South Carolina

"Todd Bowen does a great job spreading a message that is so needed in our ever 'growing', nutritionally starved, and complacent society."

-Andrew Odom
tinyrevolution.us

"My favorite parts about HIGH SPEED HEALTH are the simple, real-life anecdotes it provides. They implement quick fixes that lead to massive results over time."

-Shane Danaher
IRONMAN tri-athlete

"This is literally the Dummies' Guide to Fixing Your Body! What I love about Todd's book is that he provides information we can act on immediately. As someone who doesn't have time for a doctor to tell me what I should do 8 weeks later, I immediately started implementing Todd's easy strategies. Whether you're looking to spend basically no money by self-healing, or seek holistic treatment from the most effective specialists, this book is for you. Buy it now or stay sore."

-Zack Miller
Founder, Hatch

For my parents,
Peggy and Bucky Jr.,
who showed me the true meaning
of resilience and hard work.
Thanks, I love you.

Table of Contents

Friendly Disclaimer

The material in this book is for informational purposes only. My case was extreme. Everything in this book worked for me. I cannot guarantee that all the approaches in this book will work for everyone, as each person's individual circumstances are unique.

I became passionate and obsessive about finding as many ways possible to heal my pain. Take full responsibility for your body and choose your own path. That said, use proper discretion and consult a doctor before doing anything in this book.

HIGH SPEED HEALTH and Todd Bowen expressly disclaim responsibility for any adverse effects that may result from the use or application of the information contained in this book.

Section 1 –

How We Destroy
Our Bodies Every Day

1

The HIGH SPEED HEALTH Approach

I do not focus on providing info for athletes while they're in the gym. The world is saturated with people telling you what you should do while exercising. Your average part-time athlete only works out 10 hours a week max. I take a rare approach on how to improve quality of life and physique the other 158 hours of the week. The content I will bring you is easy-to-use, outside-the-box, and extremely effective.

"Any fool can make something complicated. It takes a genius to make it simple."

-Woody Guthrie

2

A Warning to All Inside-the-Box Thinkers

The content in this book will only work if you open your mind up to change. I'm different, creative, weird, and unique. But one thing I'm not is resistant to change.

> *"The definition of insanity is doing the same thing over and over and expecting a different result."*

> -Albert Einstein

This book is simply about my personal experience of what worked for me. It describes how I was determined to beat stubborn injuries that were caused by years and years of bad habits. I used all the techniques in this book to replenish my muscles and tendons. Eventually, these techniques allowed me to breathe life once again on the playing field, when working out, and when simply getting out of bed pain-free every morning. I'm not a doctor, physical therapist, chiropractor, personal trainer, massage therapist, nutritionist, or any other type of certified specialist. I'm simply an obsessive, athletic desk jockey who became passionate about healing injuries caused by years of bad habits.

This book outlines my failures, successes, real life examples, new habits, and descriptions of every effective practice I've learned and used (over the last 4 years) to become pain-free. These new habits and practices are what worked for me. Take all of my content for what it's worth. My focus is to provide a fresh new perception of today's rat race, as well as shortcut information that helped me heal my pain and prevent future injuries.

HIGH SPEED HEALTH will provide plenty of strategies so you can do something every single day that will get you closer to your goal of becoming pain-free. You're trying to make up for years and years of repetitive strain. In order to even begin counteracting that, you need to take a fierce approach against changing your daily habits.

I've poured blood, sweat, and tears into this research for the last 4 years. I was determined from day one and I'm 100% confident that this book will make the world a healthier, happier, and better place.

Thanks for your interest in HIGH SPEED HEALTH! It's going to be an unreal ride!

Todd Bowen

Free Report

Thank you for purchasing my book.

As a special gift, go download my FREE report on how to decrease pain when you run.

You can download it at www.highspeedhealth.com/freereport.

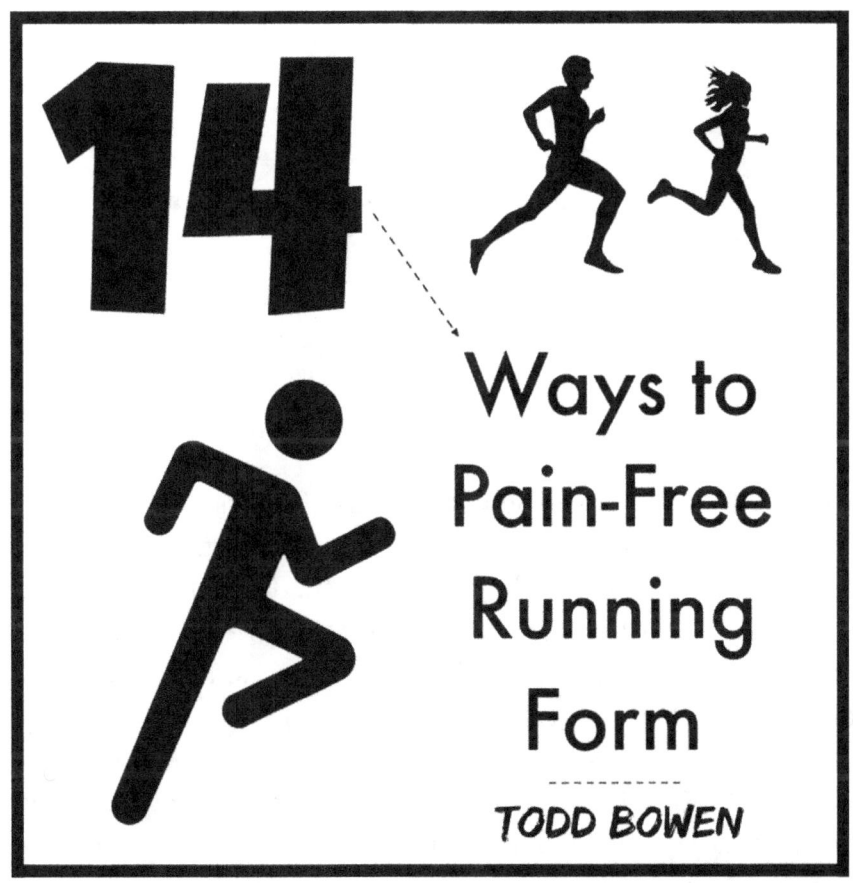

Go get it at www.highspeedhealth.com/freereport.

3

HIGH SPEED HEALTH -
A Formal Introduction

"The need for change bulldozed a road down the center of my mind."

-Maya Angelou
I KNOW WHY THE CAGED BIRD SINGS

Welcome to HSH! I've spent hundreds of hours on research and physical therapy throughout the last 4 years, battling an invisible injury that no doctor could figure out. I finally took it upon myself to become as healthy as possible, from many different angles, to defeat mind-numbing pain. During these 4 years, I've attacked and corrected every bad habit I could think of.

HIGH SPEED HEALTH is not about being perfect 100% of the time so that successes run out or burn out. The idea is to find a happy medium that is still a major improvement over our past ways. A very attainable goal would be to eliminate as many bad habits as possible, reducing muscle stress and pain, therefore increasing quality of life and physique.

On average, someone who works out 5 days a week probably works out around 10 hours a week max. That sounds great. The question is, what are they doing to live a healthy lifestyle the other 158 hours in the week they're not exercising? For most of us, 40 or more of those hours are spent sitting at a desk while gravity constantly compresses all our bones, muscles, and tendons straight to the point of pain. I've been through countless sports, hits, falls, fouls, surgeries, accidents, and illnesses. Regardless of all that, the most destructive thing I've ever done to my body was sit at a desk full-time for 10 years.

We're desk jockeys living in a rat race. Sitting at a desk and repetitive strain injuries will take a major toll on our existence. But that's only if we let it.

I wrote this book with the intention of teaching people how to take more responsibility for their own bodies. I want them to wake up feeling pain-free, energized, flexible, fast, and strong every day. I wrote it with the most basic, non-medical terms possible so any athlete can understand them. I got tired of waiting for weeks at a time to get an appointment with a doctor or specialist, only to spend 10 minutes with him/her telling me a bunch of medical terms that made my head spin. I got tired of spending thousands of dollars to see multiple physical therapists who had no idea where to begin finding the sources of my pain. I finally realized the only person that was going to figure this out was me.

What I'm not:

- Doctor
- Physical Therapist
- Chiropractor
- Personal Trainer
- Massage Therapist
- Nutritionist
- Any other kind of certified specialist

None of these specialists have experienced the extensive damage themselves that sitting for long periods of time can cause. So how can they truly know what we're going through? They might know what it does, but they haven't witnessed it firsthand to the extent that I have. The bad news is that most of the people listed above take an outdated approach to healing pain. That is, if they take a direct approach towards it at all. Each of these doctors/specialists take one angle towards fixing something. They never communicate with one another about a patient's file or history, unless the patient himself relays the info between them. They even bad-mouth each other to the patient often. They're more concerned in building their ego than they are with the patient getting a well-rounded diagnosis and treatment.

What I am:

I'm a life-long athlete and fitness enthusiast who pounded a desk, 40+ hours a week, for 10 years. I've found ways of self-healing that no doctor would ever imagine telling his patients. I was faced with a mind-numbing and physically excruciating battle against an invisible enemy. I became passionate and obsessive about body awareness and self-healing. For the past 4 years, research and physical therapy have basically become a part-time job of mine, 20 to 30 hours a week, in addition to my full-time job. I've learned much faster, more direct, and less expensive ways to self-heal compared to what these old school doctors/specialists would suggest.

It's amazing what the average person can do and learn when they focus and put their mind to something.

A person cannot do *EVERYTHING* they put their mind to.

However, I'm a firm believer that a person can do *ANYTHING* they put their mind to.

4

Injuries and Bad Habits

*"If you think adventure is dangerous, try routine.
It is lethal."*

-Paulo Coelho

We all have fires burning in our bodies. I refer to injuries sometimes as fires. You know where it's burning, but you have no idea where or why it started, much less how to fix it. You don't care if you ever find out where or why. You just want the fire put out. You just want the injury to stop hurting.

I'm 37 years young. Up until a couple years ago, I spent my adult life knee-deep in multiple bad habits, without knowing the repercussions they'd cause.

These bad habits included, but were not limited to:
- Heel striking when running
- Excessive numbers of reps during weightlifting workouts
- Rarely stretching

- Lack of proper hydration
- Excessive amounts of caffeine
- Poor nutrition
- Bad form when exercising
- Bad posture when sitting, standing, driving, and laying down
- Repetitive stress/strain

All of the above, and then some, contributed to every muscle in my body to be overly tight, compressed, and unhealthy. Just because someone is exercising or lifting a weight, doesn't mean they're taking a well-rounded approach to good muscle health and fitness. If a muscle is tight, compressed, and dehydrated, you can do all the squats in the world. It's just going to make things much worse. In addition to proper mechanics, there are many other essential pieces to the puzzle.

Think of it like this. Imagine if you could look underneath the skin of an athlete and see one muscle. On one hand, you have an 18-year-old athletic kid. This muscle is very flexible and hydrated. Imagine it as a rare piece of meat (an uncooked steak for example). It's very fluent and red (with proper blood flow throughout).

On the other hand, you have a 33-year-old part-time athlete who sits at a desk all week (with bad posture). This person's muscle used to look exactly like the 18-year-old kid's muscle, but that was 15 years ago. For the last 15 years, this person has practiced all of the same bad habits I did. Today, this 33-year-old's muscle looks like a dried up leather belt. It still works, but not efficiently. It's shorter, tighter, slower, dehydrated, compressed, and colorless (lacking proper blood flow).

If it lengthens at all during a static stretch, it'll hurt like hell first. Second, once the stretch is over, it'll go right back to the same length it was before the stretch. Sure, the muscle still works, and it's strong, but it's not nearly as reactive as the 18-year-old's muscle.

A longer muscle is a quicker muscle. Which, in this case, is the 18-year-old's muscle. The 33-year-old's muscle may be stronger, but it's much more unhealthy and compressed. It's slower and shorter. Muscles are attached to tendons. Tendons are attached to bones, very often at a major joint area, like a knee. When the 33-year-old's muscle is shorter, it puts extra strain on that tendon. This leads to incredible pain all around that joint, not only where the tendon is overexerted. These tight muscles pull on tendons more since they're too tight and inflexible, therefore inflaming tendons and areas around major joints.

How many times have you heard a person say something like...

"I can't run anymore because I'm too old."

Or, *"I hate running."*

Or, *"I can't play sports that require jumping because I have bad joints".*

Very often, the people that say these things are only in their 30's, or even late 20's!

Unless they've suffered some sort of freak injury or trauma (torn ligaments, irreparable tendon damage, broken bones, lack of carti-lage in a joint, or spinal disc deterioration), chances are this person could simply be suffering from muscles that are too unhealthy and compressed.

I refused to accept the fact that I was too old. This book will provide stories and examples of every successful decompression practice I used to get back to more than 100% of my previous athletic abilities. Not to mention, it will tell how I got back to the point of waking up pain-free every day, after years of chronic pain.

5

Four and Functional

"If people sat outside and looked at the stars each night, I'll bet they'd live a lot differently."

-Calvin (of Calvin and Hobbes)

I've been an athlete my whole life. With a physical education teacher for a mom and a five-sport father, I was swinging a golf club and shooting a basketball soon after I started to walk.

Before we can understand where we are going, let's take a look back and understand where we came from. As young children are in their first few years of life, they are very functional in everything they do. Have you ever paid close attention to a young child (as young as 18 months old) squat down to pick up a toy? Their form is amazingly good for someone who has never been told how to do a squat, or much less even understands what most words even mean yet. They even hang out in that squat position for minutes at a time playing with that toy, like it's their job. A lot of adults can't even bend over to tie their shoe without having to sit down first.

Better yet, pay close attention next time a little guy takes off running down the sidewalk (3 to 5 years old is the best). His arms are smoothly swinging with proportion. Look at his body from a side view. His entire body from the ankles up is a straight line that's correctly leaned forward with a grade between 5 to 10 degrees as he runs. His core is engaged, but he's not hinged at the waist at all. His feet are not heel striking, nor is he running on his toes. It's a comfortable combination between the two. Finally, he's looking straight ahead, not down at his feet or the ground (which would lead to massive neck issues in the future). Check out the below pictures that show a couple little guys with the good, natural running form I described above.

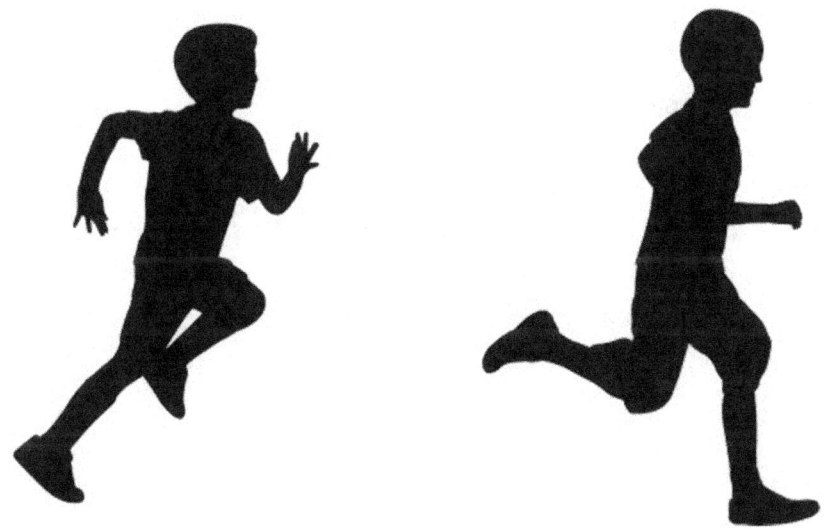

My brother-in-law is an accomplished Ironman tri-athlete and my sister is a Half-Ironman tri-athlete. My nephew is now a 5-year-old who's an accomplished 1-mile fun run racer. An 8-minute mile has never been so underrated. Watching him run is a beautiful thing. It's not because his parents jam his tiny brain full of running tips and techniques. It's quite the opposite actually. The little guy instinctively runs with such good form. It's all for fun and his parents just run next to him in these 1-mile races because, well, he's only 5. Yes, his running style is energetic and care-free partly because all his little muscles and bones are young and fresh. That's one thing we cannot totally control about ourselves as adults. I use the word "totally" because we actually can control it partially if we invest time and money in the latest good muscle health practices. I'll get into plenty of this later in the book. But the fact is that time goes on and things grow old. However, in large part he runs so effortlessly because he's doing everything functionally and correctly. Now that is something we can always control as adults. It won't be easy, but it's very attainable and realistic. Nothing great was ever accomplished without some sort of sacrifice or hard work. In this case, it'll take both of those. Not to mention patience, determination, focus, creativity, and an open mind.

You will hear me use the word functional often. I, myself, define functional as "the exact way things are meant and supposed to be done." There's no cheating on form, no maxing out, and it doesn't mean doing as many sloppy reps as possible in a certain amount of time. All those things are great if you're trying to beat your friends' times or number of reps in workouts. But the downside is this will leave you in pain with loads of unnecessary muscle soreness for days. To me, the word functional means solid form no matter the movement. Functional is sitting in a chair correctly with the proper lumbar curve in the lower back. Functional is bending over to pick up a child while using your legs, instead of your back. Functional means injury-free.

Muscles should be prime and pumped after a workout, not incredibly sore and destroyed to the point where you can barely walk or get out of a chair. In my opinion, those extreme workouts should only be done by the experts (professional athletes, tactical military, first responders like firemen and policemen, etc, etc). You'll notice that none of these studs I've mentioned will be found sitting at a desk 40+ hours a week. They're constantly moving, active, and on-the-go.

That's where we are very different.....the part-time athlete who sits at a desk full-time. We're desk jockeys living the rat race. Day in, day out. It doesn't matter how positive-minded and grateful we are, or even how much we love our life. We need to step back and re-evaluate exactly what we are doing to (and how much we are destroying) our bodies on a daily basis.

6

Perception Check - An Average Day in the Rat Race

repetitive strain injury (noun)
a condition in which the prolonged performance of
repetitive actions causes
pain or impairment of function in the tendons and
muscles involved

-Google

Here's an average day. We rush to work in the morning, crouched up tightly in the seat of our car, getting mad about every little stunt someone else pulls on the road. Stand by for a later section on "The Physical Effects of Mental and Emotional Stress." Then, we sit for 4 hours staring at a computer screen while gravity bears down on our bones at a crushing rate per second that everyone underestimates.

Then, it's lunch time. Awesome, we get to go and release some stress. We do 1 of 3 things. We might go running. Let's say we run

3 miles. Let's also say each of our strides is 3 feet long. There are 5,280 feet in a mile. You guessed it. If each of our strides average 3 feet long and we ran 3 miles, we took about 5,280 steps of pounding our feet into the concrete with every ounce of body weight we have on top of them. Man, I hope we wore some decent shoes with some life left in the sole. Or, I hope we're not a textbook heel striker. If we are, chances are that shin splints have already gotten to us. If not, they will soon, and they suck. Speaking from experience, been there, done that. Horrible pain. It takes a lot of patience and hard work to get rid of them. You basically have to stop running completely and focus on strengthening your calves through weight training or physical therapy like it's your part-time job. Then, you have to correct your running style completely, unless you just want the shin splints to come back. Striking your heel first when you run transfers all the secondary impact to your shin (which is a very bad thing). But striking your mid-foot or fore-foot (pose running) first puts that same secondary impact on your calf (a good thing) and alleviates unnecessary pressure on your shins.

Second option, say we're really hungry today and just want to go eat. We go out to a restaurant and eat so much food that it could feed a small family. Why did we eat that much? Because we're stressed about work, money, family, relationships, life in general, you get the point. Food tastes great when we're stressed. It's comforting and it takes our mind off of things. We get back to our desk in a food coma, even more tired than we were when we left before lunch.

Or finally, we might go to the gym at lunch. There's no time to stretch before or after the workout because lunch breaks are typically only an hour. We start our workout. Every tight muscle that's accumulated since we woke up that morning, that's right, it's working overtime with every rep we do. Sure, our legs are getting stronger from those squats we're doing, but our lower back has been tense since an hour after we sat at our desk this morning. It doesn't hurt while we're doing squats because it's tight past the point of pain. Plus, our legs are burning from the squats so we're thinking about that first. We think our lower back is fixed, but there are multiple layers on top of layers of muscle in our bodies. Just because something doesn't hurt or doesn't feel tight, it doesn't mean we're being functional. It could be so deep that it's inside our pelvis. There's no way we can stretch it because of how deep it is, plus we don't even know exactly where it's located. But that's not the worst of it. Everything is connected in our bodies one way or another. Everything. This muscle deep in our lower back is pulling our glut tight, which then passes strain just over our hip joint to the quads in the front of our leg. Our quads are then pulling at the tendons all the way down at our knee. These tendons are overexerted and rubbing against a bone (which is very bad). It causes tendonitis.

We take a week off from physical activity and try the old R.I.C.E. trick each day on our knee (but our knee is the effect of the pain, not the cause). Rest, ice, compress, and elevate. It works! Our tendons in our knee don't hurt anymore. We can't wait to be active again. Guess what? That lower back muscle deep inside our pelvis is still tight (the cause and primary source of the pain). Our hips are still tight too. Our knee feels great, but we don't realize our quads are still tight and we don't even know where our glut starts or ends. We try running. A half mile into it......crippling tendonitis instantly comes back in the same knee.

Time to go back to work for the afternoon of another 4+ hours of bodily destruction by gravity and a lack of ergonomics. You guessed it, sitting at a desk. But now we're dejected and frustrated that we can't run. Our knee cap feels like it's going to rip off with every step we take walking to the printer. Then an old friend shows up. His name is work and he's ready to stress us out all over again. Our desk chair is some beat up, old thing that's been around the office for years longer than we have. It's padding is broken down so there's minimal support, the arm rests are probably way too far apart to keep our elbows on in the right position (causing neck and shoulder pain), and the chances are that the back of the chair is way too deep for us unless we're taller than 6'8".

Finally, it's 5:00 pm. If we don't work late today, we have 2 to 3 hours to do what we want. That's right, only 10% of the day. Then another 2 to 3 hours to run errands, eat, and prepare for bed or the next day. Then we get to go to sleep. Hopefully we're a good sleeper and know how to release from our work day to relax, because we get to wake up 8 hours later and do it all over again.

7

Body Awareness

resilience (noun)
1. *The ability of a substance or object to spring back into shape.*
2. *The capacity to recover quickly from difficulties: toughness.*

-Google

The human body is one of the most complex systems we'll ever encounter. Yet, some people know more about cars then they do about their own body. The capability of humans to heal muscles and maintain good muscle health is far beyond what the average athlete understands, or can even imagine.

There are plenty of people out there to tell you what you "should" do. Doctors, specialists, coaches, trainers, therapists, friends, smart people, idiots, you get the point. But no one knows your body like you do. Take everything these people say into consideration, decide quickly if it's right for you or worth your time. This is called accurate discernment (which is an incredibly powerful asset). Don't harp on it. Either work it into your routine or don't, then move on immediately. Take full responsibility for your own body.

> *"By trying to please everybody, you'll end up pleasing nobody."*
>
> -Mark Cuban
> *Owner, NBA's Dallas Mavericks*
> *Self-made Billionaire*

Don't worry about what other people think if you don't take their advice. Just say thanks and look at them like they're weird. They'll second guess themselves. Don't get into a debate with them. It's a waste of energy. Who cares? Or just tell them thanks and that you'll start doing exactly what they said. This way they'll stop bothering you about it. But then, go do what you want. Don't be a sheep and follow the herd just because they tell you to.

> *"By the way, what have you done that's so great? Do you create anything, or just criticize other's work and belittle their motivations?"*
>
> -Steve Jobs
> *Co-founder of Apple Inc.*
> *Visionary and Creative Genius*

It's time that we learn to take full responsibility for our structural health upon ourselves. Primary Care Physicians, Orthopedic Specialists, and Chiropractors are amazing people. They're incredibly smart. They know how to fix one of the most complex organisms that exists. Humans. However, it's not like the old days. Doctors used to be genuinely concerned in helping all their patients get healed as soon as possible. Doctors don't treat patients anymore, they treat numbers of patients. Instead of concentrating on spending ample time with and helping patients complete their rehab successfully, they are focused on how many patients they see. The latter is a much higher number than the former. I don't believe it's the doctors' faults. Maybe it's the larger corporations that oversee them who stack the appointment books full of back-to-back patients, maybe it's the lack of doctors and the surplus of patients in our world today. Who knows.....the answer is irrelevant. What matters is, if we don't take responsibility for our own bodies, no one else is going to start doing it for us.

It's easy to tell a doctor that our knee hurts. It's not easy to attack the source of that pain. It's even harder to locate the source of that pain. There could be hundreds of reasons as to why a major joint like a knee is hurting. Most of them are not located inside the knee, even though that's where the pain comes out, and that's where the doctor takes the x-rays.

Let's look at an average timeline of someone getting injured, then treated.

Primary Care Physician

We get hurt or start to notice pain. We go see our primary care physician. The primary care physician probably won't refer you to physical therapy. He probably wants an orthopedic specialist to do that. The PCP refers you to an ortho.

Orthopedic Specialist / Orthopedic Surgeon

You call to make an appointment that day with an ortho, but he's booked 2 to 6 weeks out.

For the next few weeks, you spend every day and night in pain, trying to exercise around it without making it worse. You're unhappy and constantly disappointed that you're in pain and can't get in to see the ortho sooner.

Then, it finally comes. Appointment day. The orthopedic specialist's assistant takes x-rays on what the doctor thinks could "possibly" be the issue, but the ortho still hasn't even seen you yet.

The ortho finally comes in and talks to you for 10, maybe 15 minutes if you're lucky. He prescribes 800mg per day of an anti-inflammatory. As if we don't have enough wrong with us right now, like 800mg per day of anything is going to make our body a cleaner place, or make us feel any better over the long-term.

You ask if surgery is an option. Unless you've suffered one of those freak injuries I mentioned earlier (torn ligaments, irreparable tendon damage, broken bones, lack of cartilage in a joint, or spinal disc deterioration), the ortho is probably going to recommend against surgery. First, you never want to cut anything in your body unless it's the last resort. There's always, always a chance that the surgery won't correct the injury. Second, surgery ain't cheap. Third of all, the ortho probably won't even be sure what the source of the pain is, so he won't want to cut anyway.

I'm not saying people should stop going to their primary care physician or orthopedic specialist, far from it actually. I'm trying to inform them on how they can be more prepared to get an effective, most-efficient use of their time when they go to an appointment.

When you're researching your injury, begin using the image search option on your favorite Internet search engine (I use Google). There should be a way to search images as opposed to web sites. If your search engine of choice doesn't have this option, switch to one that does. Start searching body parts that hurt and find images and diagrams of the muscle composition of that body part. Print them out. Get familiar with the muscles surrounding this body part and try to figure out which ones are tighter than others. This is called body awareness. I'll talk more about that later. For now, start taking an approach to stretching or releasing the tight muscles. I'll also cover plenty of different methods on how to do this later. You don't need to get too in-depth while studying the muscles and diagrams, or become an expert in anatomy. Just start to get an understanding of how different muscles and joints work. This image search option should become one of your most utilized assets, next to hot yoga and your foam roller (we'll cover those very soon too).

I showed up to an ortho appointment one time with diagrams like these printed out.

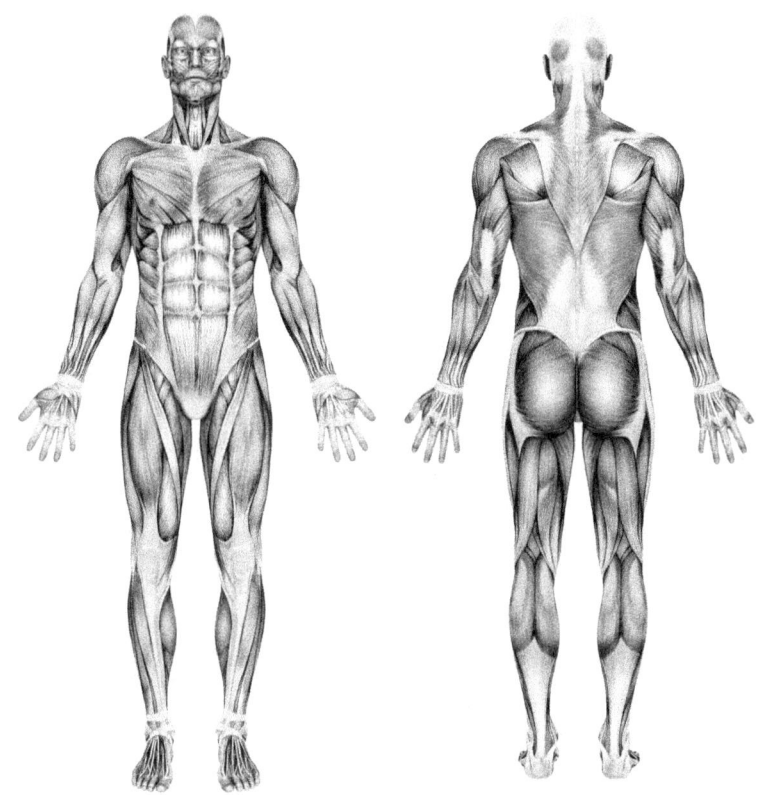

Except, I had used colored markers to draw all over my diagrams. I would shade in different muscles that were my problem areas. I'd shade in joints that were hurting me. I'd also take a black marker and draw arrows that described where I could feel the muscle tension pulling. The ortho was even more inclined to help me, because of my intensity in trying to figure out the source of the pain. He was much more interested in my case because I gave him clearer, more detailed info to work with.

Also, show up with a list of questions. The small amount of minutes you have with an ortho go by fast. Don't risk going in there and forgetting to ask a question just because you didn't have it written down. You'll be waiting at least a month for your follow up appointment.

Finally, one thing an ortho won't hesitate to recommend is physical therapy.

Physical Therapy

Your ortho writes you a prescription for PT, 2 to 3 times per week for 6 to 8 weeks (for example). By the way, your health insurance probably doesn't cover physical therapy, and the rate is a lovely $30 to $60 per hour.

I may have gotten a couple bad eggs in my experience with physical therapy. I'm sure there are PT's out there that really know their stuff. Even so, the reason for pain in a major joint (like a knee) could be from hundreds of different sources. Why go to a physical therapist and have some kid tell you what they "guess" you need to do? They're trying to put out a fire with an eye dropper. Sure, it might be helping a little, but there are much faster, less expensive ways to get this accomplished than old school medicine practices. The idea is to change your daily habits by making them as holistic and healing as possible.

8

My Take on Human Muscles

Human muscles are incredibly fascinating if you take a few minutes to learn about them. Let's look at a specific muscle. Take the hamstring, for example. Many people think the hamstring is only one muscle. Actually, depending on how you look at it, the hamstring is made up of 3 different major muscles. These include the bicep femoris, the semitendinosus, and the semimembranosus. Don't worry, when it comes to medical terms, that's as technical as I'll get throughout this whole book.

But let's look even deeper than that. Take just one of those muscles, or any other specific muscle in the body, and understand that there are multiple layers on top of layers of muscle intertwined and on top of each other. When we were young 18-year-old kids, our muscles were so fresh and potent that they never really got tight. Even before or after we exercised or played sports, we didn't need to stretch at all. Then, time, overuse, repetition, bad form, lack of hydration, and bad nutrition started to set in as we got older. The first layer of muscle that will be affected is the very bottom layer (closest to the bone). It's the first layer that reacts when our mind is made up to make a movement. But that is so deep that we can't even feel it unless we are getting some type of deep tissue massage. The top layer that we mainly think about is the last layer to react. It's also the last layer to get tight. There are multiple layers in between the top and bottom layers.

Think of each of these different layers as a rubber band. All of the layers put together are like dozens of rubber bands wound up into a symmetrical ball. You can't take all these rubber bands apart at the same time. You have to take them off one at a time. Layers of muscles work the same way. You can't stretch them all at the same time. You can only stretch one or two layers at once. When those layers become flexible, then you can move on to the deeper, tighter couple of layers.

I prefer doing each stretch longer than the average user would do. Let's compare a muscle to a 2 inch rubber band. If you stretch the rubber band out to 6 inches for 10 seconds, then let it go, it's going to go right back to 2 inches long. However, if you stretch that rubber band to 6 inches for 10 minutes, then let it go, it'll be longer than 2 inches. I'm not saying to do a static stretch (like touching your toes) for 10 minutes straight. I'm just saying I take a much different approach to stretching muscles, all of which I'll talk about on the upcoming pages.

There is no x-ray, MRI, or CT scan machine in existence that can detect tight and unhealthy muscles. The composition of a healthy muscle looks the same as an unhealthy, tight muscle. The only difference looking at the x-ray is that the unhealthy one may be shorter than the healthier one. It's up to the user to increase his/her body awareness and pinpoint the problem areas. Fix one area, another one will tighten up. That's life. Now fix that one. Then the next one. Or for those inside-the-box types, consider the only other alternative. Just keep living life the way you are, in pain with limited range of motion and flexibility.

9

Muscle Compression

"Many a false step was made by standing still."

-Fortune Cookie

There are many factors to take into consideration when talking about long-term muscle health. Basically, any time that you are contracting muscles to gain strength and/or stability, they are being compressed. For someone who doesn't practice any muscle decompression techniques at all, years of daily compression will lead to smaller, tense muscles. It will also lead to a continuous decline in performance and a constant increase in pain.

Examples of Muscle Compression:

Sitting
Driving
Lifting weights
Running
Lying on a couch
Sleeping in bed

Jumping
Landing
Emotional stress
Mental stress
Walking

    Take your average athlete who lifts weights, runs, drinks water, and eats somewhat healthy. Just because they do all these things, it doesn't mean they're taking a well-rounded approach to take care of their muscles.

Section 2 –

Healing Your Current Pain from Repetitive Strain Injuries

10

Intro – Muscle Decompression Part 1 - The Latest in Professional Muscle Health Practices

The next eight chapters will give descriptions of the professional services I've tried. I've listed these chapters in alphabetical order. A lot of them focus on muscle decompression. All of them focus on muscle health. Remember, just because we exercise, it doesn't mean our muscles are healthy. There needs to be a balance of many different variables (hydration, nutrition, stretching, muscle decompression, cardiovascular training, and strength training just to name a few).

11

Active Release Techniques

My (IRONMAN tri-athlete) brother-in-law suggested I try Active Release Techniques. A.R.T. is a practice where a therapist strategically uses his hands and fingers to put pressure on a patient's tight, troubled area. He then instructs the patient to do a certain (active) movement. During that movement, the therapist's pressure on the patient actively releases the tense muscle a little bit with each movement. Each movement is usually done numerous times. My appointments lasted either a half-hour or an hour.

My A.R.T. therapist prides himself on providing a "good hurt." The movements are painful. However, the pain was gone and I had increased range of motion every time I got up from his table. He was also very knowledgeable in a wide variety of topics including Exercise Science, Sports Medicine, and Nutrition.

I was very satisfied with the results I got from attending multiple A.R.T appointments. They were relatively inexpensive too. On average, it was about the same price per visit as my chiropractor.

12

Acupuncture

I don't have anything against specialists who provide acupuncture as a secondary service. For example, sometimes you'll see a chiropractor (primary service) who also provides acupuncture (secondary service). However, I'd highly recommend finding someone who primarily focuses on acupuncture. It makes a huge difference. I've tried both. One day I was referred to a lady who focused solely on acupuncture and herbal healing solutions. After I went to her for the first time, I'll never go to anyone else. It completely changed the way I looked at acupuncture, as well as healing as a mindset.

First of all, from the second I stepped in the door, the overwhelming smell of a peppermint scent helped me detach from my stressful workday. The scent helped me begin to focus on healing immediately. I still hadn't even checked in yet.

After I had a seat in the waiting area, I notice there is a very small water fountain strategically placed on a table. There are small metal chimes floating in this fountain. The soothing sound of running water splashing gently into more water was extremely calming. That running water would make those metal chimes bump into each other occasionally, making a soft chiming sound each time.

Then, I check out the magazine stand. I grabbed one of the coolest, most outside-the-box magazines I've ever read. It was a magazine that focused on yoga, healing, and natural living. At this point, I had practiced hot yoga for 3 years now and it never once crossed my mind to look into reading a magazine about it. Thanks to that appointment, I've checked out many issues of that magazine since then and learned a ton from it.

All of these things helped me leave a stressful workday and transform into a very relaxed state. All that and I still haven't even talked to the acupuncturist yet. Then I get called into a room. She spends about 15 minutes asking me tons of questions, very concerned about taking the best approach possible to help me heal quickly. I also brought in diagrams and questions on paper about my pain. She was very interested in learning about my specific case, while not jumping to any conclusions or taking anything for granted.

Finally, she puts the needles in. Then, she leaves me to the most relaxing 30 minute nap I've ever had. Especially impressive, considering I was laying on a flat, cushioned table and not on a bed. I wake up with a very refreshing and surreal feeling.

I was so relaxed on the drive home, it was mind-blowing. I no longer cared about many of my small problems. It was like seeing life in a whole new light. As far as my larger problems, I now saw them as small hurdles. I didn't worry about them nearly as much. The time that I did think about them, I was trying to figure out a solution to alleviate the problem as opposed to stress about it. My whole perception about everything changed just from that single appointment.

You'll pay more money to go to a healer who has acupuncture as their primary focus. However, I highly recommend it. My appointments with this acupuncturist took an extremely unique approach to healing and the results were incredibly satisfying.

13

Body Memory Recall

Throughout the course of life, we go through many types of injuries. These injuries can be physical, mental, or emotional. When we don't express or exert these injuries fully, these injuries stay hidden in our physical bodies. We all have a body memory that is very fresh and functional as a child (refer to my earlier Chapter 5 "Four and Functional" for more info). As time goes on, this body memory accumulates physical, mental, and emotional stress. These stresses lead to an invisible muscle tension. This muscle tension pulls our bodies out of alignment and into a very non-functional state. This is invisible and very tough to diagnose, much less correct.

Body Memory Recall is a very deep muscle release practice that a healer does by hand. It's the deepest and most excruciating pain I've ever experienced in my life. However, the pain is temporary and would be completely gone by the time the healer took their hands off of that area. Every time I got off the table, my flexibility and range of motion were improved drastically.

Like all of my favorite muscle decompression practices, B.M.R. takes a very holistic approach to living. It's expensive, but well worth it. Without Body Memory Recall, I'm convinced I'd still be waking up with pain in both knees every day.

14

Chiropractic

I've heard every excuse in the book when it comes to why people don't go to chiropractors. Our bodies get knocked in and out of alignment all the time, whether we get adjusted by a chiropractor regularly or not. The more our muscles are compressed, the easier it is to get out (and stay out) of alignment.

Bottom line: Go to the chiropractor, people. Please! You'll thank me later. Trust me. The human body is a terrible thing to destroy.

But don't just go to any chiropractor. Ask around and try to get referred to one that has a similar active background that you have. For example, I like to run, swim, weight train, and push my body to its limits. Therefore, I asked as many athletes as possible who the chiropractor was that they used. I ended up going with a chiropractor who was referred to me by a tri-athlete. The chiropractor is also a dedicated tri-athlete himself. He's one of the top swim/bike/runners in the state of Virginia in his age bracket. This gives him an extensive understanding of how to correct and align athletes' bodies properly. He views life from the same perspective most of us do, the durable part-time athlete who also sits at a desk often.

My chiropractor also does Active Release Techniques as a secondary practice. This is a huge benefit having both A.R.T. and chiro under the same roof, at the same appointment, at the same time.

Going to a chiropractor is definitely going to improve your quality of life and physique. There's no question about it. It'll open new doors and give you the capability to be even more effective in your movements.

15

Massage Therapy

I don't go to your typical massage therapist. I just don't have the mindset to relax on a table where someone you don't know is giving you a sensual massage (when you're paying money for it). I don't have anything against normal massage therapy. It's just not for me.

Massage therapy is a good muscle decompression method. It soothes skin, relaxes muscles, and increases blood flow. All of this essentially leads to faster muscle recovery. However, I'm all about the fastest results possible (like you haven't guessed that by now). I just think there are many more effective practices out there that give quicker results.

16

Muscle Activation Techniques

Just because someone is strong and in shape, it doesn't mean all of their muscles are activated and working properly. Muscles can become deactivated over a period of time with bad habits and repetitive strain. It doesn't mean the muscle doesn't work at all, it just means the muscle doesn't work all the time when it's supposed to. Basically, the muscle isn't working up to its full capability.

This is where Muscle Activation Techniques are very helpful. M.A.T. is a very technical practice where the healer puts a certain amount of pressure (not very deep) on a specific area of the muscle. He only needs to hold the pressure there for a couple seconds. This will allow the muscle to activate more efficiently when it's supposed to.

My experience with M.A.T. was a good one. When lying flat on the healer's table for the first time, I had an awful external rotation with my left leg and foot. Basically, my right foot was pointing up towards the ceiling and my left foot was pointing towards the wall on the left side of the room. M.A.T. helped me to correct that quickly (within a few weeks of 2 sessions per week).

However, I went to M.A.T. early in my recovery phase. At that point, I had no idea how many compressed, unhealthy muscles I had to tackle. It ended up taking a lot more M.A.T. appointments to get results because of how tight my muscles were. M.A.T. would've been much more effective for me if I would've waited until I was farther along in my recovery with looser muscles.

17

Rolfing Structural Integration

Rolfing Structural Integration is a form of bodywork that reorganizes the connective tissues, called fascia, that permeate the entire body (www.rolf.org/about). It approaches the body as one complete system, opposed to multiple different parts.

My experience with Rolfing SI has been great. The "Rolfer" uses their hands to release the tension of muscle fascia. This allows a more efficient use of the muscles that are surrounded by the fascia. Sometimes, the pressure is single-point. Other times, the Rolfer uses two hands simultaneously. Sometimes, the client is resting passively during the technique. Other times, the Rolfer will have the client do active movements while they are Rolfing.

I'm a huge fan of Rolfing SI. It has improved my flexibility and posture tremendously.

18

Summary – Muscle Decompression Part 1 - The Latest in Professional Muscle Health Practices

If I had to do my recovery all over again, knowing what I know now, I'd go to more Rolfing and Acupuncture in the beginning for muscle release. Those 2 practices got a lot deeper into my deepest layers of tight muscles. Then, I'd go to more Active Release Techniques and Muscle Activation Techniques towards the end of my recovery. I would have gone to the Chiropractor the entire time during (and after) my recovery.

19

Intro - Muscle Decompression Part 2 - Self-Healing and Self-Maintenance Practices

The next twelve chapters will give descriptions of the self-healing practices I've used. I've also listed these chapters in alphabetical order. Experiment with them and see which ones work for you. Use multiple self-healing practices at the same time to force multiply your performance and results.

20

Compression Clothing

Ok, it's about to get tricky here for a minute. Bear with me. I've been talking for a while about how muscle compression is a bad thing. However, wearing high-quality compression gear over your muscles is a good thing. It supports muscles by keeping them in place where they're supposed to be. This essentially causes them to be more efficient, more functional, and reduces muscle fatigue and damage. This will essentially help lead to muscle decompression. Compression clothing also increases blood circulation throughout your body, allowing muscles to recover more quickly.

I've been wearing high quality compression gear on and off for the last couple years. My brand of choice is 2XU (www.2xu.com). There are other brands that I've heard are good, but I've never used them. Any compression gear that gets good reviews in the tri-athlete community will probably do the job well.

2XU has two different lines. One is called "compression" that is made for wear during sports and exercise. The other is a "recovery" line that is made for post-workout wear or while sleeping. The recovery line is an even tighter fit that helps your muscles recover more quickly, whether you are sleeping or just wearing it around the house.

   Do not go for the cheaper compression gear that the bigger companies mass produce and sell for $20 to $30 per short. Save your money and spend it on something more high-quality. You might as well not even wear compression gear. This cheaper gear feels tight and it's moisture wicking, but that's about it. It's not a graduated fit that increases blood circulation and supports muscles correctly like 2XU does.

21

Ergonomics

Learn all about proper ergonomics. Your body will thank you for it, trust me. Pay close attention to my upcoming Chapter 36 about about Posture in my FORCE MULTIPLIER METHOD.

I'm not going to sugar coat it. People who sit at a desk with bad posture need to understand that they are destroying their bodies. When you're destroying something 5 days a week, 40 hours per week, it won't take long before things start to decline and fall apart. It's a huge issue that's going to lead to more pain, doctor visits, a decrease in quality of life, future surgery, etc, etc. Who knows what could happen? The possibilities are endless.

Sitting at a desk with proper ergonomics will not only decrease everyday pain, but it will improve your efficiency, flexibility, energy, and range of motion in the gym and on the playing field. People need to learn that they can fix bad ergonomics by taking a few small steps and implementing them into their daily routine. It's not going to be easy to break out of these bad habits. However, it's very attainable. Plus, it's your only option aside from a life of pain.

22

Foam Rolling

Go buy a foam roller, today. Trust me. It'll be your best friend in your quest for a pain-free life. Foam rolling allows you to use gravity to give yourself a deep tissue massage. It will pay for itself within the first hour that you use it. It costs less than a one-hour deep tissue massage from a certified massage therapist.

For those who've never foam rolled before, get the long cylinder completely made of foam, it's the softest one out there and a good beginner level tool. This roller will only last for a certain amount of usage. That's just the way it is. You should get at least a few months out of it, even if you use it a lot.

Eventually this first foam roller will get beat up and resemble a firm pillow more than a circular foam roller. When this happens, you can either get another one of those or graduate to an intermediate level roller. The intermediate roller I recommend is my favorite, the Triggerpoint Grid Roller (www.tptherapy.com). It looks like a big PVC pipe with a thin layer of cushion all the way around the outside of it. If I had to make a choice to only use one wellness tool for the rest of my life, it would be this foam roller. It comes in a couple different lengths. I'd get the longer of the two options, unless you want to travel with it or keep it at your desk at work. Both of which I do, so I also have one of the shorter versions.

Once you get really good at foam rolling and you're ready to take it to the next level, graduate to a foam roller called the Rumble Roller (www.rumbleroller.com). It's an intense tool that gets really deep into your muscle tissue, deeper than any standard massage you've ever gotten. There are a couple different firmness levels and a couple different lengths.

If you're super experienced in foam rolling, you can take it to another intense level. Buy a 4" diameter PVC pipe from a hardware store. Be very careful when you start using a PVC pipe. There's no padding at all so there's much less room for error. I recently began using a PVC pipe, but only after tons of experience with padded foam rolling.

Generally speaking, the less padding on a foam roller, the deeper it gets into the layers of muscle. Another general tip, rolling quickly on a foam roller will mostly improve blood circulation and stretch the top layers of muscle (closest to skin). The slower and more patient you roll, the more you will get the deeper layers of muscle to react (closest to bone).

Foam rolling is an art. It's not an exact science. We've all got unique bodies with different amounts of muscle tension in different areas. I've spent hundreds of hours on a foam roller within the last four years. I know, I'm crazy and weird. That ain't the first time I've heard that. Tell this dude something I don't know. It's all perspective, I consider the alternative of where I'd be if I never used one. I'd definitely, without a doubt, still be waking up with pain in both knees every morning. Even if I used it a minimal amount, I'd be nowhere near where I am today. I'm back to 100% of my previous athletic ability. Now I'm focused on improving that another 20% at the ripe age of 37 years young.

Don't roll around on it fast. The idea is to go very slow. Start off by letting the roller rest in one place, allowing the tight muscle to stretch and "melt" around the roller. Then, once you've started to get results in that one spot, you can slowly roll as the muscle is stretching. Every time you get to a spot that really hurts, stop on it. Let that tight spot stretch and watch the results snowball from there.

There are many different angles to take on different body parts. For example, when rolling your calves, you'd think you only need to do the back of them. That will help, but you won't get the full results unless you roll the outside of your calves as well. That's a muscle too, and it's directly connected to the back of your calves. If you roll one angle of a muscle and get it loose, the angle you don't roll will remain tight and eventually pull all of the loose muscle tight again.

Let's look at another example, the back. It's great to just lay flat on the roller and go up and back a couple times. But you also need to turn slightly to each side and do your lats. After that, take it a step further and do your sides (or obliques).

And after you do your whole back, think about your abdomen. How many sit-ups or crunches have you done in your life? 1,000? 10,000? More? Now think about how many times you've decompressed your abdomen. Once? Twice? Never? I told my chiropractor I rolled my abs and how much of a liberating feeling it was. He said he never thought of doing such a thing. It was then that I realized, I either really was weird and obsessive, or I really was on to something.

How many pushups have you done in your life? And how many times have you gotten the deepest layers of your chest muscles massaged or decompressed? You get the point by now.

I can hear you now, it's a good thing I live by myself. I know, I know. There's no way anyone would be able to contain themselves by watching me do self-healing on a foam roller. I'm like a hippie on that thing. But if that's what it takes, then that's a small price to pay for me being successful. I attack everything from the bottom of my feet all the way up to my forehead. Yes, I even release facial muscles with it. It's an incredibly liberating feeling. Head, face, and neck muscles get very tight too, you know. With a creative and open mind, you can foam roll anything.

My chiropractor said it best. I've come back from something that most guys just don't make it back from. They give up sports early in life. They stop working out. They take pills, drugs, turn to alcohol, etc, etc. I committed myself to figuring this out. I'm determined to never quit until I'm successful, or dead. Whichever comes first. Life's good and anything's possible. Anything.

Back in the low points of when I was getting crushed by chronic knee tendonitis, I would wake up on a Saturday morning and not want to get out of bed. It was so depressing. I'd make myself get out of bed, then turn on the TV. I'd lay on the floor in front of the

TV with a foam roller for hours. I'm talking about 6 to 8 hours per day on some weekends, 2 to 3 hours per night during the week. Obviously, I wouldn't roll constantly during these hours-long sessions. I'd take breaks. But still, it was brutal, both mentally and physically.

These days, I still keep all 4 different flavors of foam rollers at my house. Which one I use, and when, just depends on how tight the muscle is and what I'm trying to get accomplished. Don't make the same mistakes I did. Take care of your body and avoid unnecessary injuries and pain. Refer to my upcoming section on my FORCE MULTIPLIER METHOD for quick and easy ways to prevent future pain.

23

Hot Yoga

People, please, please, please. If you've never done hot yoga, try it at least a couple of times. It'll give you a whole new understanding of your body awareness and what needs to be corrected. Not to mention, it's a great way to clear your head and relax. For new clients, most studios offer a trial period of unlimited visits for the first week. These are usually cheap, $20 or so for the whole week, which is a very good price.

Hot Yoga is one of the most relaxing things I've ever done. Up to 105 degrees of pure hotness. I know what you're thinking!

"That sounds so miserable."

"It's too hot."

"I'd get so sweaty."

"I can't afford it."

Blah blah. Waah waah. Try it. Trust me. It's not much more intense than spending a day outside on a hot, humid beach. You get used to it quickly and you won't regret it.

The goal of taking these hot yoga classes is to heighten your awareness of what's going on in your body. Our biggest problem is we don't know what the root of our pain is, so it's nearly impossible to fix. We need to take an approach to healing all of our muscles, our entire body simultaneously. Instead, we tend to focus on healing a certain joint because it hurts. That joint, let's say a knee for example, could hurt because of a tight muscle in our hip. We'll never think to stretch a tight muscle in our hip if we're so concentrated and stressed on the pain in our knee. In my opinion, hot yoga is the best way to approach healing your body as a whole. The other best way? It's fueling your body with proper hydration and nutrient-dense foods. Combine hot yoga with proper hydration and healthy food as fuel, watch your results multiply quickly many times over. We'll get into plenty of this later in the book.

Back to hot yoga, don't give up after just one session. I felt terrible during and after my first session. I knew I had just begun my journey to counteract years of repetitive strain. So, I had to be patient. As terrible as that first class was for me, I knew there was potential healing and results ahead of me by continuing hot yoga. My second and third sessions were a whole different story. Every move came much more easily. I felt better physically and mentally. I slept better and I woke up with more energy. Better sex is also a benefit of taking hot yoga. The results began to come very quickly after my second and third classes.

Set a realistic goal of taking your first 3 or 4 classes within 10 to 14 days. That's not too tough. Substitute hot yoga for running or weightlifting if you have to. Trust me. Hot yoga is an incredibly powerful practice.

If you ever feel pain in class, remember these two things. First, back off slightly. Pain is not a good thing when practicing. Back off and be patient. Second, remember to breathe. Don't hold your breath. Breathe in deeply through your nose. Breathe out slowly through your mouth.

Also, go ahead and skip the whole room temperature yoga thing. I'm not saying that doesn't help a person relax or give them results. But, I am saying that the hot temperature in hot yoga exponentially expedites the amount of time it takes for your muscles to get warm, loose, and have an increased blood flow. Therefore, your muscles stretch much more quickly and easily, giving you faster results and faster muscle decompression.

24

Inversion Therapy

Also known as.....hanging upside-down like a bat, by your feet. This practice was introduced to me by my Body Memory Recall healer. I practice this on and off. The most I'll do it is 5 minutes at a time, 3 times per day. We spend all of our lives with gravity bearing down on us. By practicing inversion, it slowly works against gravity and counteracts its effects on us. It's a relaxing way to get a full body stretch, simply by hanging there. Also, like when wearing high quality compression gear, inversion improves blood circulation. Recently I've started wearing my compression gear while doing inversion, which multiples the results. It's incredibly relaxing as you can feel blood flowing through body parts that normally lack circulation while standing straight up.

There are a couple different set-ups you can choose from. One of them is basically to buy a pull-up type bar that goes inside a door frame. It then extends to hold itself up inside the door frame. Then, you can get some inversion gravity boots. They don't really look like boots. They secure tightly around your ankles and contain a hook on the outside. After grabbing the bar with your hands, you throw your feet up and hook your ankles to the bar. Only thing left to do is let go of the bar with your hands, extend your upper body towards the floor, hang, and relax.

The second option is to purchase an inversion table. It takes up a lot more space in your house, but it's much safer and more secure. Being the single guy living in a bachelor's pad apartment, I opted for this option. It's tucked away against the wall right when you walk in, but I'm not exactly your better homes and gardens type of guy. I'm more into high human performance and quality of life, compared to what people think of me. I know ladies, I know, it's much easier to be a guy. Lol.

25

Lacrosse Ball

Another way to attack and release a tight muscle is to use a lacrosse ball. You can get them for about $3 each at your local sporting goods store. It sort of takes the same approach as a foam roller, allowing you to use gravity to give yourself a (free) deep tissue massage. Instead of using a foam roller, a lacrosse ball should be used when you really need to get deep into a very stubborn layer of muscle that's been overused and tight for a long period of time (years, for example).

Another good thing about the lacrosse ball is it's about as compact and convenient as you can get. It's great for travel. One time, I flew from Virginia to California, with a layover in Tennessee. We didn't switch planes in Tennessee, so I was in the same seat for about 6 hours. I'm 6'3" tall. After about an hour into the flight from Tennessee to California, one of my hamstring muscles tightened up so much, it reached a point of numbness and my leg fell asleep. I didn't have many options other than getting up and walking around for a minute on a crowded plane, which may or may not have improved my situation. Then it hit me. My backpack was under the seat in front of me. What was in there? Aw yeah. My lacrosse ball.

Talk about dumb luck. I just happened to leave it in there instead of in my checked suitcase. I took it out of the bag and placed it on my seat underneath my leg. Putting it right on the tight hamstring muscle allowed me to use gravity to stretch it, just by simply sitting still. It was an excruciating stretch, but 5 minutes later, the muscle wasn't tight and my leg felt fine.

You can also use the lacrosse ball while lying on the floor or leaning against the wall. The lacrosse ball is very small, so sometimes you'll need to elevate the ball in order to get enough pressure on the muscle to begin releasing it. In this case, you can put a yoga block on the floor (or wall) and put the ball on top of the yoga block. Don't roll around on the ball, at least not at first. Just let the ball rest in one place, letting the tight muscle stretch and "melt" around the ball. Then, once you've started to get results in that one spot, you can roll the ball slowly into another tight spot and start over again.

26

Liquid Calcium Magnesium Citrate

<u>*Disclaimer:</u> I've said it before and I'll say it again. I'm not a doctor or any other type of certified specialist, so do not take my advice as if it's good for everyone. I'm simply telling my real-life stories about what worked for me. That said, Liquid Calcium Magnesium Citrate is an off-the-shelf supplement that can be bought at your local health food market.

My Active Release Therapy guy recommended this to me. It was during an appointment with him a couple years ago, when I had some serious issues going on due to excessive numbers of reps while weightlifting. I'd also had a lot of stubborn tension in my neck, back, and shoulders due to years of overuse, repetitive strain, and bad posture while sitting at a desk.

He told me that a lot of long-distance tri-athletes use L.C.M.C. After a few days of use, it puts your muscles into a very relaxed state. It removes toxins from your system, making you feel much less sluggish. Your muscles become very pliable and less support-ive, but that's a good thing. You want this because it allows you to get faster results when decompressing muscles (while stretching, foam rolling, hot yoga, etc.).

Use Liquid Calcium Magnesium Citrate with caution. Start off at a lower dosage than what's recommended on the label until you get used to it. It cleans out your system and also acts as a laxative (if you know what I mean). Another reason to use caution is that it will put your muscles into a very relaxed state, essentially making your muscles temporarily weaker. You won't be able to lift the same weight you normally do. Also, if you get to the point where you take a lot of it, your muscles won't support your body as well as they normally do, even while doing common movements like running or walking.

If you take these cautions into consideration, Liquid Calcium Magnesium Citrate is a great way to multiply your muscle release results. My dad is a retired truck driver who plays golf every other day. I recommended L.C.M.C. to him. He was skeptical at first, but he's gotten great results from it and now he's a huge fan. It costs about $14 and that bottle will last me about a month. It's most effective when taken on an empty stomach. However, make sure to drink at least one full glass of water after taking it.

Some tri-athletes just use L.C.M.C. for about a 10 day cycle. Others use it year-round, but at a much lower dosage. Magnesium is a mineral that is found in many vegetables. It's up to you how much to take. Take responsibility for your own body and figure out what works best for you.

27

Percussion Massager

A friend who's also into creative wellness practices turned me on to this item. It cost me $100. I got it from a techie store at the mall. It's a handheld massager that has 3 different speeds. It penetrates deep to relax and soothe tense muscles, also improving blood circulation. Improving blood flow is a huge asset in muscle recovery and decompression, if you haven't noticed by now.

28

Pre-heat Therapy

I actually learned this from one of the bunk physical therapists I went to. It was one of the few helpful tips I got from that guy at a painful $60 an hour. Now that I do all my physical therapy on my own, I work pre-heat therapy into my routine often. I just use your average heating pads that you can get at any drug store. All of my problems are usually identical (or close to it) on each side of my body. I'm pretty big into being symmetrical, whether it comes to self-healing or strength training. Therefore, I'll usually use two of these heating pads at the same time.

I'll do pre-heat therapy in order to warm up the overused, stubborn, and tight muscles. This heat will increase the blood flow in the affected area. If you're using the heating pad on a leg, foot, or arm, wrap something like a belt, shoelace, or yoga strap around it so it's nice and snug. I'll heat it for about 10 minutes until the body part has plenty of blood circulation, even a decent sweat on the skin is good. Then, I'll jump on a foam roller and roll the warm area out for a while. This practice, yet again, is another way to exponentially multiply your results when working towards muscle release (decompression).

29

Self-Massage

Since I started to get experience and results in releasing tense muscles, I've learned how to give myself a self-massage. The idea is to put pressure on one spot with your thumb, just hold it there and let the muscle slowly stretch and "melt" around your thumb. After it's been in that one spot for a while, start to slowly move your thumb around. Remember to go very slow or else the muscle will not be pliable and results will be hard to come by.

P.S. This may not work at all if you aren't hydrated properly and/or you have a poor eating routine. To get the best results with any of these decompression methods, make sure you are fueling your body properly with water and a nutrient-dense, real food eating regimen. I can't stress how important this is enough. Plenty more on this to follow later in the book.

30

Static Stretching

I know, static stretching sucks and it's frustrating. But once I followed these practices in this book to increase the overall muscle health in my entire body, I actually enjoy static stretching now. It may take months, even years to get there, but consider that compared to your only other option. That is, living the rest of your life in pain on your current training plateau with a glass ceiling that limits your results.

31

Summary – Muscle Decompression Part 2 - Self-Healing and Self-Maintenance Practices

Combine as many of these practices together at once to exponentially multiply your results. Here's an example of what I'm doing right now for muscle decompression wellness.

Compression Clothing – I sleep in recovery compression gear every night. I sometimes wear active compression shorts under my swimsuit when I'm playing beach volleyball games and tournaments. When running, I either wear high compression socks or calf sleeves. I also wear a short sleeve compression shirt and shorts when I'm doing hot yoga and strength training. In addition to increasing blood circulation, this tight fitting compression gear helps me keep better posture and form.

Ergonomics – I've been known to sit on a balance ball while at my desk, use an ergonomic keyboard, and keyboard tray. The keyboard tray slides the keyboard closer to my upper body. This way, I don't have to reach forward to type (which would overextend my shoulders). I'll get into this more in my next section, The HSH FORCE MULTIPLIER METHOD.

Foam Rolling – Hours and hours and hours of it. Remember, you're trying to make up for years of tension, overuse, and repetitive strain injuries. Be patient and don't let frustration get the better of you.

Hot Yoga – Anywhere between 1 to 5 times a week (depending what sport I'm playing or other activities I'm doing at the time)

Inversion Therapy – 2 to 3 times per day, 5 minutes each time

Liquid Calcium Magnesium Citrate – 1 to 2 tablespoons per day followed by a glass of water

Percussion Massager – As needed

Pre-heat Therapy – As needed

Self-massage – Every day, multiple times, very often, and whenever I can (whether I'm relaxing, working at my desk, driving, etc.)

Free Report

Don't forget to pick up my free report.

It's only available to those who purchased HIGH SPEED HEALTH.

You can download it at www.highspeedhealth.com/freereport.

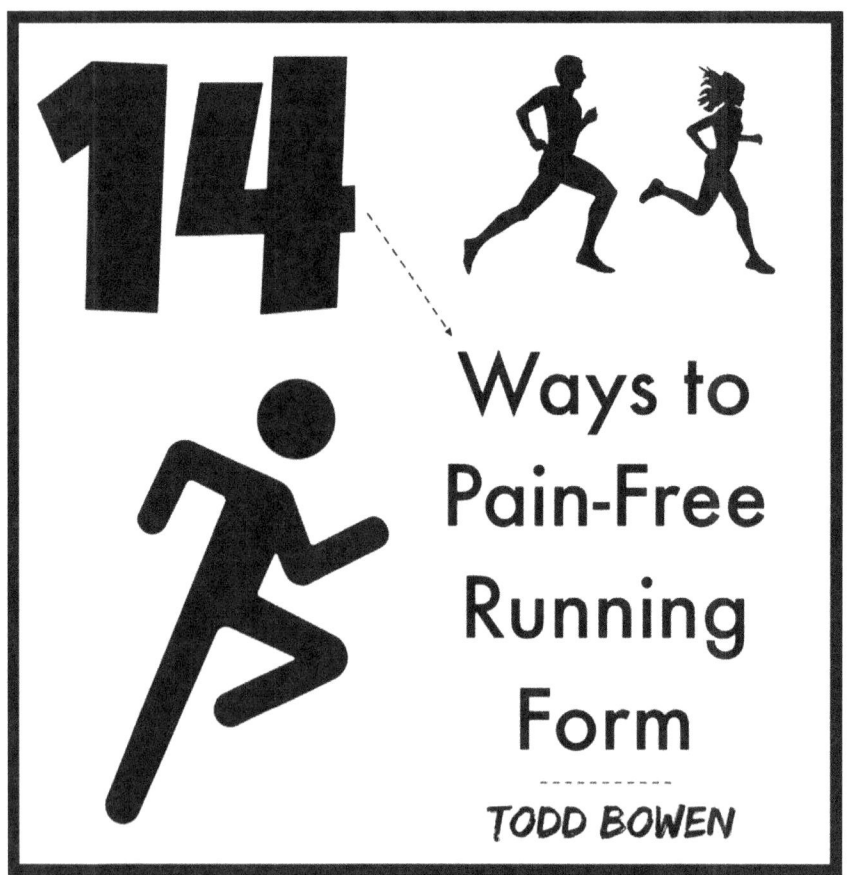

Decrease your pain by going to www.highspeedhealth.com/freereport.

Section 3 –

Preventing Future Repetitive Strain Injuries

32

THE HSH FORCE MULTIPLIER METHOD

By now, you've noticed that I do not focus on providing info for athletes while they're in the gym. The world is saturated with people telling you what you should do while you exercise. Your average part-time athlete only works out 10 hours a week max. I take a rare approach on how to improve life and physique the other 158 hours of the week. The content I will bring you is easy-to-use, outside-the-box, and extremely effective.

You may have heard the term "force multiplier" before. In case you've never heard it, a force multiplier "refers to an attribute or a combination of attributes which make a given force more effective than that same force would be without it." (http://en.wikipedia.org/wiki/Force_multiplier)

For example, let's say you could heal 1 injury within 4 weeks just by improving your posture while you sit. Or, you could heal that same injury within 2 weeks by improving your posture and increasing your daily intake of water at the same time. Or, you could heal that same injury within 1 week by improving posture, increasing water, and taking hot yoga classes. These are examples of force multiplication.

How many force multipliers do you apply to health and wellness? And how many of them do you apply simultaneously?

This method will tell you about my 5 most important (and often overlooked) force multipliers.

1. Hydration
2. Nutrition
3. Portion Control
4. Posture
5. Breathing

The goal of THE FORCE MULTIPLIER METHOD is to make you less susceptible to future repetitive strain injuries. By taking an all-around look at our health and wellness, this method will ultimately lead to improving your quality of life and physique as a whole.

Here we go...

33

Hydration – Force Multiplier # 1

It used to be a rule of thumb to drink 8 glasses of 8 ounces of water per day (64 ounces total). Nowadays, recommended levels have skyrocketed to (drinking) 1 ounce of water for every 1.5 pounds of body weight. To figure this out, take your body weight and divide it by 1.5. For example, I weigh 185 lbs, so I'd drink about 123 ounces of water per day. That's a huge difference compared to the old rule of thumb's total 64 ounces. Drinking 123 ounces is probably too much for me on a cool rest day. But the only downside to drinking too much water is going to the bathroom often. However, contrary to popular belief, that's actually healthy. So it's really not a downside at all. Just because water is going straight through your system doesn't mean it's not doing its job. It's still doing you a lot of good by cleaning out your system that short amount of time that it's in there.

Bottom line: It's up to you to figure out how much water to drink in a day. There are many different variables when trying to figure it out. Each of our bodies and daily activities are so unique. Just take these 4 factors into consideration:

1. **<u>Temperature -</u>** A day spent inside with an air conditioner will require a lot less water than a day out on the beach in the middle of the summer.

2. **<u>Physical Activity Level -</u>** Rest days require a sufficient amount of water, but not as much as an intense workout day.

3. **<u>Body Weight -</u>** The more you weigh, the more water you need to drink, simple as that.

4. **<u>Amount of alcohol, caffeine, and sugar consumption -</u>** These 3 guys are the biggest enemies of hydration. Take them in moderation as much as possible. Also, whenever you consume them, make sure you drink some water either before or after. It'll help with digestion. Also, the alcohol, caffeine, and sugar will have less of a dehydration effect on your body.

Here's my normal, everyday morning routine. The first thing I do is fill up a 32 oz. bottle of filtered water when I wake up. Filtered water is great. It's very clean and the filter can even make bad water taste good. The only problem is, it can filter out the minerals that muscles need for recovery from strength and cardiovascular training. So I'll add a very small shot of a liquid mineral supplement to my water. It makes the water taste lighter and even better. You can find it at your local health food store. But look at the nutrition label. Don't get liquid minerals that contain sugar. That defeats the whole purpose of hydrating yourself.

Now back to my morning.......I'll be done drinking that 32 oz. bottle by the time I leave the house at 7:30am. I know! I'm so crazy!

How? I keep it within arm's reach when I'm in the shower. I know, I know. It doesn't sound like the most sanitary concept, but I've never gotten sick from it. That's because I drink so much water... duh. Just don't keep it down low in the shower. Keep it up high, somewhere on a ledge or a towel rack. Then, I don't need to drink any water for at least the next couple hours. The rest of the day, I just drink water as I need it, depending on the temperature outside and my physical activity levels.

Alert - most important paragraph you'll read all day

Think about it like this. When you went to bed, you probably went to bed dehydrated, so you wouldn't get up in the middle of the night to use the bathroom multiple times. Totally understandable, good sleep is underrated. Then, you sleep for eight hours breathing constantly which depletes even more of the hydration in your body. Then, the first thing you do when you wake up is get into a steamy shower. You guessed it, breathing in steam from the hot water depletes your body's hydration even more. This is why people are exhausted when they get to work in the morning after a good night's sleep. Then, they drink a cup of coffee because they're "tired". People don't realize the reason they are "tired" is because they're dehydrated. Guess what? Your energy from the caffeine is going to be very short-lived. Why? Because there's no water in your body to take the caffeine through your system. You haven't been properly hydrated for at least 12 hours by now.

Outside-the-Box Thoughts

1. **Don't drink your calories.** Sports drinks are OK during exercise and after exercise, but use moderation and be very mindful of how much sugar they contain. In regards to fruit

juice, soda, coffee, and tea....take some time off from them and replace them in your day with an extra glass of water. Your energy level WILL go up after a few days, guaranteed. Alcohol....you worked out hard all week, reward yourself and enjoy it. But if you drink a lot of it within a few hours, work in some water too. It'll make your morning-after much easier.

2. **Eat your water.** Fresh and steamed vegetables contain a lot of water and minerals. Or, cook them in olive oil. It's high in unsaturated fat. Unsaturated fat is a good thing for athletes. It's necessary for building muscle. Unsaturated fat is also an energy source. The more vegetables you eat, the less water you can get away with drinking.

3. **Drink more water in the hours leading up to your workout, as opposed to during or just before.** This outside the box thought is courtesy of Shane Danaher, IRONMAN Triathlete. An IRONMAN is an endurance race that is 140.6 miles long. It's made up of a 2.4 mile swim, a 112 mile bike ride, and a 26.2 mile run. It takes time for water to get absorbed into your system. Unless it's a long endurance workout, the water you drink during your short workout is just helping keep your throat from being dry on the way to your stomach. By the time the water is absorbed, your workout is over. This isn't necessarily a bad thing, because water is good for post-workout muscle recovery. It's just a good reason to make sure you ALSO drink pre-workout. The more water you drink before, the less water you'll need and the more energy you'll have during your workout.

"I can easily tell after a workout when I didn't drink enough water, not DURING, but well before a hard session. It totally kills my recovery."

-Shane Danaher
IRONMAN Tri-athlete

21 Day Hydration Challenge

If a person sticks with something every day for 21 days straight, it's much more likely to become an everyday habit.

1. Try increasing your water intake the minute you wake up for 21 days. I realize that 32 ounces by 7:30 am is extreme, but I weigh 185 pounds. If you're the same size as me, start off at half that to get used to it, 16 ounces. If you never drink water in the morning, you can even start off with 8 to 12 ounces and you'll probably see a big difference. If you're female, y'all need a lot of water for reasons I won't even act like I understand. But a more important factor is that you're smaller, so start off with just 8 ounces and work your way up to 12 or 16.

2. Give up ALL caffeine (coffee, soda, sugar-free "energy" drinks, etc.) for the same 21 days.

You CAN drink alcohol during this challenge. I strongly believe in rewarding yourself (in moderation) from a hard day's work, but try to drink some water around that same time.

If you complete this challenge successfully, at the end of the 21 days you will have more energy, a faster metabolism, improved mental clarity, less muscle soreness, and quicker recovery times. You'll feel better all-around throughout your whole day. If not, you can call me whatever bad name you want. Three years ago, I gave up caffeine 100% and I haven't had it or craved it since. I'll probably never go back to it, unless it's a safety concern (like driving at night on a long road trip).

34

Nutrition – Force Multiplier # 2

"Let food be thy medicine and medicine be thy food."

-Hippocrates

If you remember anything from this section on nutrition, remember these 3 most important words (please!):

"EAT. REAL. FOOD."

Basically, invest in quality, nutrient-dense, organic foods. Don't eat just because you are hungry. Think of it as fueling your body for optimal performance.

In my opinion, real food is either an animal, a plant, or it grows on trees. For example, real food consists of (but is not limited to) quality organic red meat, chicken, fish, seafood, vegetables, fruits, eggs, nuts, and seeds.

Real food is something that people ate back in the days before there were grocery stores, like the cavemen for example. Cavemen didn't eat oatmeal, yogurt, everything bagels, or drink coffee and soda. I'm not saying these are the worst things in the world. But, I am saying there are other options that are much cleaner and better for you.

I'm also not saying you have to eat real food all the time. Just try to increase your amount. For example, if you eat real food 60 to 70% of the time, that's much better than eating it 25% of the time. And try not to buy anything that comes in a box or a can. True real food rarely comes packaged like that.

Keep in mind that I'm different, obsessive, weird, wild, and a little crazy! But when I hit the grocery store, here's the route I take:

Produce section
Natural foods aisle
Meat counter
Seafood counter
Dairy section
Frozen vegetables aisle (rarely, I buy fresh vegetables 95% of the time)

With the exception of the natural food and frozen vegetable aisles, I didn't go to any of the middle aisles. I stayed in one big circle around the outside of the store. I never go in the middle unless I need toothpaste, tissues, toilet paper, or anything else that starts with a "t" that's not food. Next time you go to the store, try to not even step foot in those aisles. The middle aisles are mostly full of processed foods loaded with preservatives and chemicals. That's why they don't need to be refrigerated. Go for the fresh stuff.

Produce section - Hit the produce section hard and buy a lot of green stuff! The darker the green, the better it is for you. I usually don't buy anything that I won't eat within 5 days so it doesn't go bad. And buy some of those green (sometimes they're blue) bags that keep vegetables fresh longer. They work! Plus, the more vegetables you eat in a day, the less water you have to drink. For all my haters of drinking water, that's right! Vegetables are filled with water and minerals that hydrate you in addition to the water you drink. It's a win/win!

Also, I always buy organic vs. non-organic when I have the chance. I know! So expensive! That extra $.50 to $1.00 per product is worth it. You never know what types of chemicals are used in non-organic foods these days. I've said it before and I can't say it enough, "Who puts a price on their health anyway?"

When shopping for vegetables, remember that "no-carb" is just so 2000 and late, especially if you're an athlete. Carbs are necessary for your brain, quick reaction time, and good decision making throughout your day. Vegetables contain all kinds of vitamins to give you energy and minerals to help you recover. Who wants to be a zombie all day anyway? Been there, done it. Stay tuned for Part 3 of the FORCE MULTIPLIER METHOD for tips on maximizing energy every day in simple ways people easily overlook.

Natural foods aisle – Sometimes I get olive oil, organic thin crust pizzas, dark chocolate, and other good organic sweets from here. Some of these may come in a box, but they're organic and natural ingredients, so they're legit enough for me in moderation.

Meat counter - If you're getting burger or steak, try to buy lean if you eat red meat often. If you don't eat it often, not-so-lean is OK. Consider it one of your reward meals.

Try to purchase quality, non-processed meats. Some grocery stores post a welfare rating on how the animal was treated.

Seafood counter - As far as seafood, white fish is typically the healthiest. But if not, hey, you're still eating fish. It could be a whole lot worse. You're in good shape.

Dairy section – I used to buy organic whole milk. Yes, it was worth it. It tastes much better and cleaner than the cheap stuff. Plus, cows are terribly mistreated throughout the majority of the country. When buying non-organic milk, you're rolling the dice as far as what you're putting in your body.

Nowadays, I don't drink milk at all. I'm more of a vegetable and fruit smoothie type, blended with coconut water.

I get organic, cage-free brown eggs. Fry them in either olive oil or coconut oil. That's good stuff right there.

I get cheese. Don't worry about it being fat-free as long as you're active. Plus, the fat (from fat-free cheese) is removed by adding chemicals (toxins) that are not natural.

Don't buy yogurt, just don't do it. It's got way too much sugar, especially for breakfast.

Disclaimer: *Many people will argue that some (or most) dairy is not "real" food. Again, the purpose of HIGH SPEED HEALTH is not to be perfect 100% of the time. The purpose is to constantly improve and evolve our lifestyles into an equation that equals high human performance.

Frozen vegetables aisle - As far as vegetables go, frozen vegetables are a lot better than no vegetables at all. Obviously they aren't as nutritious as fresh (never frozen) vegetables, but this isn't a perfect world. If it was, there would be a farmer's market every 6 blocks instead of a convenient store.

Healthy Dessert Option

Instead of peanut butter cups, candy, or chocolate bars (all of which I grew up on), substitute natural, organic dark chocolate. The higher the % of cocoa, the less sugar it contains. For example, I usually go for the 88% cocoa bars. They only have 10 grams of sugar total, but you won't need the whole thing. One bar lasts me 3 days. They usually come in small squares so I can divide them up easily. Very inexpensive, about $3 bar. You can find these on the natural foods aisle at your local grocery store or health food market. Anything less than 5 grams of sugar at a time will just flush right out of your system quickly as long as you're hydrating properly with water.

Another tip, try to start eating fruit as a dessert occasionally. Fruit contains sugar too. It's a good way to reward yourself, while not suffering the energy crash you'd get after eating a high-sugar dessert (such as candy or anything containing processed sugar).

Homework Challenge

Next time you're at the store, try taking my route. See if you can avoid buying ANYTHING in the middle aisles. Besides, the money you save from those middle aisles will be put to great use on all those organic, nutrient-dense, natural foods you're buying now.

Perception Check:

Do you enjoy eating healthy? Or do you suffer through it?

If you don't find a way to enjoy it, chances are it's going to suck. Make it fun and interesting. Temporary diets are for quitters. Instead, make it an enjoyable lifestyle change and keep improving on it every day. Longevity, consistency, and being subtle are key, not being quick and on a crash diet.

35

Portion Control – Force Multiplier # 3

I like to compare portion control to the maintenance on a car. Oil changes, refueling, and replacing tires all have different timelines in which they need to be done. If you always get these 3 types of maintenance done on your car earlier than necessary, it's a waste of time, money, and resources. If you wait too long to get maintenance done, it decreases your car's performance and becomes a safety hazard.

The same goes for eating and portion control. If you eat too early or eat too much, you're consuming calories before your body is done digesting the previous meal. Your current meal might taste great or even be healthy, but it is excess calories your body doesn't need yet. These excess calories won't digest properly or burn off easily. The outcome is feeling sluggish. If you wait too long to eat on the other hand, your body goes without the nutrients it needs and your metabolism slows down. On top of that, you're starving so you're likely to over-eat at your next meal. The outcome is feeling weak. Either way, your body isn't going to run efficiently. If you begin practicing portion control, it'll maximize your energy levels and caffeine will become a thing of the past!

The best way to maintain natural energy is to pace your intake of calories. You don't have to over-eat or under-eat, and the body has the amount of energy it needs. You're already going to eat every day, change your ways to be more effective at it and watch your energy levels shoot through the roof.

These are not the old days where 3 meals a day were the standard. If you want to take care of your body and get the best results possible, you need to practice (proper maintenance by) eating smaller meals more frequently throughout the day.

On an optimal day, I'd describe my eating regimen as 3 small/ medium sized meals plus 2 small snacks per day. On an optimal day like this, I really won't even get hungry or tired at any point in the day. That's because I spread out my caloric intake as evenly as possible. But notice I said "on an optimal day". Don't get me wrong, occasionally I will knock down 4 or 5 pieces of pizza with ice cream for dessert. You have to reward yourself sometimes.

Anyway, my point is that it's okay to do what you want at times like these. Enjoy yourself. Reward yourself. You don't need to be 100% strict about nutrition and portion control every day, far from it actually. You'll have plenty of time to make up for it Monday through Friday. I'd describe my portion control ratio at about 80/20. 80% of the time I eat very healthy with appropriate portions. 20% of the time I loosen up, relax, reward myself for hard work, eat more than I should, or eat whatever I want.

So, start off small when thinking about portion control (no pun intended, kind of). If you eat better and practice strict portion control 5 days a week with 2 cheat days, it's much better than practicing it 0 days a week. However, I'm strongly against entire cheat DAYS. I'd suggest cheat MEALS instead (just a personal preference). After an entire cheat DAY, you'll wake up feeling very tired and sluggish the next morning.

Let's do the math on my 80/20 rule. Say I eat 4 to 5 meals/snacks per day. Multiply that by 7 days. The answer equals between 28 and 35 meals/snacks per week. For simplicity's sake, let's grab 32 out of the middle. If I eat 32 per week, 20% of 32 is 6 or 7 meals/snacks. So I'll take those 6 or 7 cheat MEALS per week and spread them out across the 7 days. That's how I practice moderation with portion control.

What is portion control? How do I measure food?

In my opinion, the best way to learn about portion control is to go on The Zone (www.zonediet.com).

The Zone is legit. Aside from the food, here's what you'll need:
- A digital food scale (about $20)
- Measuring cups and spoons (plastic is fine, probably less than $5 to $7)
- About $10 to $12 in plastic containers, get 2 or 3 different sizes (medium, small, and smaller)

Here are some keys you need to know:
- THE ZONE's types of food can be briefly described as meat, vegetables, nuts, seeds, some fruit, little starch, and no sugar.

- Eat within 10 minutes after you wake up. Kick start your metabolism. Eat something. Anything, even if it is just 1 fried egg (cooked in olive oil or coconut oil) and some almonds (preferably natural almonds, not smoked or salted).
- Eat each following meal between 3 to 5 ½ hours after the previous meal.
- Ideally, you should include carbs, protein, and unsaturated fat with each meal/snack (unsaturated fat is a necessary component for building muscle). Some examples of unsaturated fats are almonds, peanuts, cashews, macadamia nuts, avocados, and olive oil.
- Eat more fruits in the morning. They contain vitamins and give you energy.
- Eat more vegetables in the evening. They contain minerals necessary for muscle recovery after exercise and while sleeping.
- Salads, the greener and darker they are, the more nutritious they are.
- Oh and eat organic foods when possible. I talked about this in the previous chapter, Nutrition - Force Multiplier # 2. I can't emphasize how much better I feel since switching over to organic. Your body will thank you for it. Organic foods are grown without the use of synthetic pesticides, chemical fertilizers, or genetically engineered ingredients. Organic foods contain no artificial flavors or preservatives.

Stop it! I know what you're thinking!

"This sounds way too complicated."

"I'm never hungry first thing in the morning."

"I'll never have time for this."

"I don't want to weigh or measure my food."

Whatever! It's all about perception. One of the benefits (in eating smaller meals more frequently) is the preparation time is shorter. For example, my typical first meal is 2 or 3 fried eggs (cooked in olive oil), a banana, and a handful of almonds. Total prep time for that is a whole 4 to 5 minutes. Also, you only have to measure food for the first 2 to 3 weeks. After that, you'll know how to estimate it without the measuring scale/cups/spoons.

The bottom line is, make it work. Be creative and find different ways to do it. It's not a sprint race to lose as much weight as you can as soon as possible. Picture it as a long, consistent marathon. Think outside the box. Don't just raise your goals, raise your standards too.

"If you don't start taking accountability of your body now,
nobody else is going to start doing it for you."

-Todd Bowen

Refer to this site for an in-depth view of The Zone: www.zonediet.com.

I've done THE ZONE for a month. What now?

Now you know what true portion control is! Graduate to Paleo immediately!

Paleo eating is clean, natural, real food. The word paleo means older or ancient (Google). The name paleo originates from the ancient times of the caveman. If the type of food wasn't around when the cavemen were here, then don't eat it. Ever wonder why there were no obese cavemen? It wasn't because they didn't have grocery stores and walked around starving. It was because all the food they ate was natural. Nothing came in a box, food wasn't mass produced in a factory, and there were no chemicals or preservatives in food.

You won't need to buy anything extra that you didn't already buy for The Zone. The only thing different is you won't go in a single aisle in the grocery store except to pick up olive oil and rice vinegar. You'll likely be eating a lot of salads. Olive oil and rice vinegar were my salad dressing of choice. Everything else is picked up in the produce section, the meat counter, seafood counter, natural foods aisle, and the dairy section. Some people think this sounds "odd" or "weird", but this is the way things are supposed to be. This is why cavemen's muscular physiques were so defined and ripped up.

Anyways, I'm just your average, hard-working athlete who takes great care of himself at least 80% of the time. I'm not a nutritionist, so if you want a more in-depth description about Paleo, do an Internet search on it. Plus, there are many different variations of Paleo. Some are very strict. Some are much more lenient. In my opinion, the important thing is you are making a solid effort to eat real food.

A very knowledgeable source on the Paleo topic is Robb Wolf: http://robbwolf.com/what-is-the-paleo-diet/

Summary - Portion Control

I've never counted a calorie in my life. I don't even count protein, carbs, or fats anymore. Could I do a better job of this if I wanted to? Definitely. Do I want to? Nope. I'd rather take that time and focus it on specializing other areas of my life further. Time is a huge asset. The argument can be made that time is a much larger asset than money.

Don't go on a diet. Make it a lifestyle. Make it taste good, fun, and interesting. Temporary diets are for people who don't want to constantly improve and get the most out of life. They'll just fall back into their old bad habits after the diet and gain that weight back.

If someone asks you about it, refer to it as your "eating regimen" or your "healthy lifestyle". At first people may look at you like you're crazy, or maybe even joke you about it. But as you get more confident, they'll realize you take it seriously and you know what you're talking about. There's been many times when someone joked me for being healthy, then later they'd become interested and ask for my help.

Even if you aren't confident about it yet, act like it. Keep talking like you know your stuff. With a little patience and determination, you will know what you're doing in no time.

36

Posture – Force Multiplier # 4

"Life doesn't get better by chance, it gets better by change."

-Zig Ziglar

No matter how good we think our posture is, chances are that it could always be better. The goal is not to have perfect posture 100% of the time while standing, walking, sleeping, and sitting. No one does that. I've been an athlete all my life, but sitting at a desk has caused the worst injuries I've ever had. Bad posture was a major contributing factor. These injuries are commonly referred to as repetitive strain injuries (also known as repetitive stress injuries).

HIGH SPEED HEALTH is built on concepts that are consistent for long periods of time, like a permanent lifestyle for example. It's not about being perfect all the time so that successes run out or burn out. The idea is to find an attainable, happy medium that is still a major improvement over our past ways.

A very attainable goal would be to eliminate as many bad habits as possible, reducing unnecessary muscle stress and pain, therefore increasing quality of life.

Standing/Walking

One bad habit I had for years and years was that I would stand with my knees locked, almost bowed backwards. I was so used to standing that way, I didn't even realize I was doing anything wrong. For the correct way to stand, check out the following image and how this guy's knees are slightly bent and relaxed, not locked. This is sometimes referred to as a micro-bend. The bend in his knees is so slight that you can barely see it, but it's there.

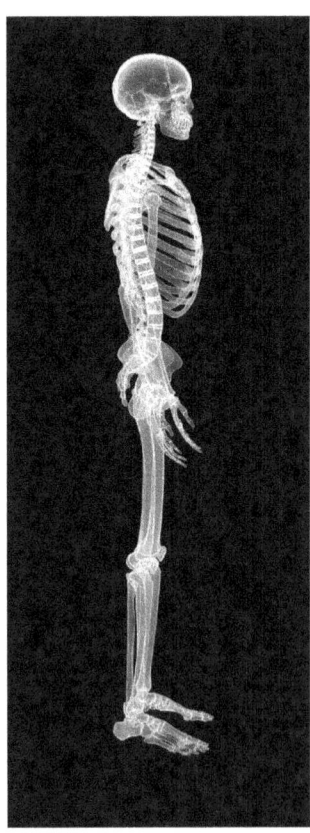

Try to stand and walk with your knees relaxed and slightly bent. At the same time, engage your leg muscles, which will be the base support of your body. Try to keep your quads, hamstrings, calves, and gluts all contracted proportionately. This will reduce tension and soreness in any one area. It'll also allow your body to move with proper mechanics, avoiding injury. Try to keep your knees relaxed and bent when both standing and walking. It'll reduce joint pain and unnecessary muscle strain significantly.

Keep a slight lumbar curve in your lower back. Keep your chest/rib cage leaned forward over your pelvis slightly. If you glance down, you should NOT be able to see your pelvis or ankles. Your chest should be blocking most of your feet. You should barely be able to see your toes though.

Keep your head directly over your upper body, not leaned forward or back at all. Balance is the key. Otherwise, this will cause unnecessary neck pain. Trust me, I know all about this from first-hand experience.

Check out the following front view of our good posture guy for good measure.

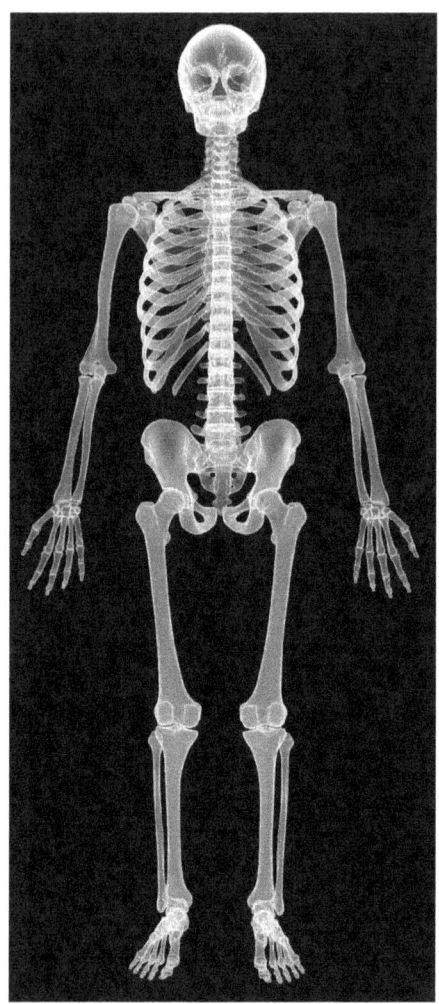

Sleeping

Our posture while we sleep is the least of our worries. Sitting, standing, and moving are far more damaging when we have bad posture. But! Sleeping with bad habits can still easily cause muscle tension issues and repetitive strain injuries. That said, if you've got an obsessive personality like me, try these helpful hints.

Sleeping on your back - Try putting a (somewhat thin) pillow underneath your knees. This will disengage your knees, relaxing your muscles from your calves all the way up to your lower back.

Sleeping on your side - Place the pillow between your knees. This will keep your legs aligned properly and reduce muscle stress and fatigue, mainly in your hips and pelvis area.

Sleeping on your stomach - Put the pillow under your ankles. This is similar to the concept of using a pillow under your knees when sleeping on your back. It disengages your knees, relaxing the muscles from your calves to your lower back. Put your feet together at the toes and let the heels fall open away from each other.

Keeping those 3 hints in consideration, I try to make sure that I don't ONLY sleep on my back, or my side, or my stomach. I change it up often. When you're sleeping, it's nearly impossible to be aware of your posture and positioning. You can try to improve it, but as soon as you fall asleep, your muscles will probably fall into the bad habits of your repetitive strain injuries. That is why it's most important to be conscious of your posture before you fall asleep.

Sitting

First and foremost, don't sit down with anything in your back pocket (especially a wallet or phone). Doing so WILL definitely knock your hip and spine out of alignment. It will also cause a major muscle tension imbalance throughout one side of your body. Once you stop sitting on your wallet or phone in your back pocket, your body will thank you for it! Trust me, speaking from plenty of experience here.

Guys, take your wallet out of your back pocket and don't ever put it back there again. It doesn't matter if it's slim or if it's a George Costanza thick wallet (Seinfeld fans know what I'm talking about here). I know, I know. Old habits die real hard. I had carried mine back there ever since I started carrying a wallet, until 4 years ago when a chiropractor told me my hip was out of alignment because of it. Ever since that day, I've switched it to a front pocket or cargo pocket and it's made a huge difference. Don't carry anything back there if you're going to sit down on it (phone, cash, tissue, anything). It will throw off your whole alignment. Ask any chiropractor about that.

Don't think it sounds like a big deal? Think about it this way. My aunt has been carrying a pedometer around lately. Last time I saw her, she had taken 8,000 steps that day and the day wasn't even over yet. Imagine the unnecessary stress, muscle fatigue/tension, and pain that 4,000 steps (with that leg out of alignment) would cause one side of your body. And that is just one normal day! Think about a day when you do heavy squats or go for a long run.

Use a Balance Ball as a Desk Chair

Using a balance ball will make you sit with better functional posture, otherwise you'll fall off of it. It will also make you engage the correct muscles. It'll increase blood flow throughout your body, including to your brain, even making you more productive and effective at work.

You're already sitting at a desk 40 hours a week. Get a bonus from it. Get a physical reward from it. Work out while you're sitting there and be more productive with work at the same time. It's a no-brainer.

I highly recommend this practice. You can start off slow, 10 hours per week out of your painful 40. I know, I know. The idea's been out there for years and people will joke you for being a weirdo. Who cares? Small price to pay. Do it and watch your physique improve drastically in a matter of days.

There are different sizes to these balance balls. It's important that you get the right height. I'm 6'3" tall and the size of the ball I use is 75 cm (just to give you something to base your buying decision off of). When sitting on a ball that is the right height, your hips should be just slightly higher than your knees. Try to focus on keeping a comfortable balance of tension between your abdomen and your lower back. They should be working an equal amount, not one more than the other. Remember, balance between your abs and your back is the key.

The average cost of a balance ball is about $20 to $22 at your local sporting goods store.

****<u>Most important thing you'll do all day that'll only take 2 minutes</u>****

Check out this image. Print a copy or take a picture of it and post it at your desk, or on your computer monitor. Put it somewhere so it's very visible and you'll see it multiple times a day. This will serve as a consistent reminder to straighten up.

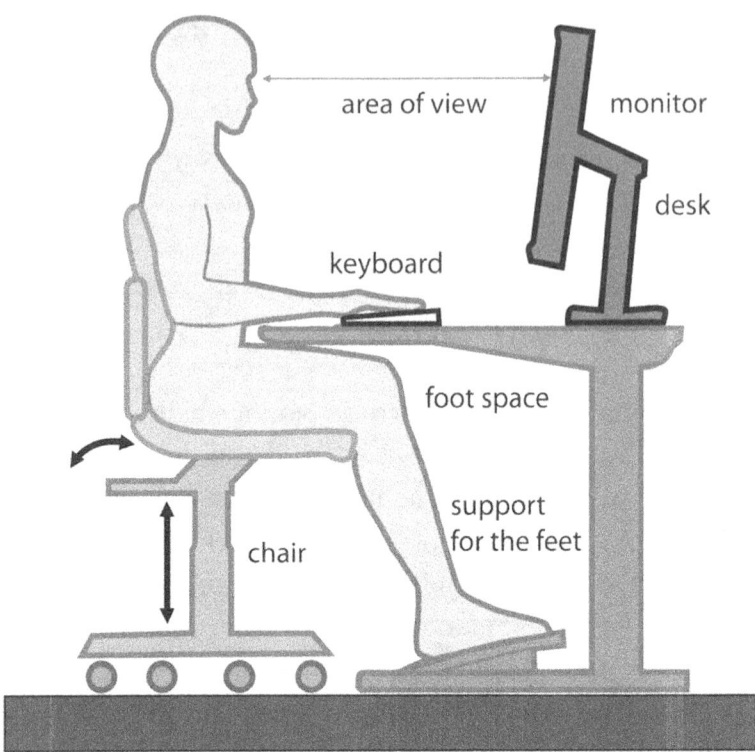

Here are some tips to help you find balance while sitting at a computer desk:

- Avoid looking down at your fingers. It will cause issues with the back of your neck/spine.
- Keep your head directly in line with your shoulders (if looking from a side view). Do not let your head drift forward or backward.
- Shoulders are back, down, and relaxed.
- Low back is arched slightly forward (also referred to as a lumbar curve).
- Legs are uncrossed.
- The top portion of your monitor should be eye-level.

- Keyboard, mouse, and desk space should be at a level that is a 90 degree angle (or a little greater) at your elbows.
- Your seat height should be so that your hips are slightly higher than your knees (when looking from a side view).
- The back of your seat should allow you to keep your upper body comfortably at a 90 degree angle with the floor.
- Your ankles should be either directly under your knees, or just slightly ahead of them. Never let your ankles drift behind your knees.
- A footrest that provides a slight degree of incline for the feet is also a very effective tool to release strain on the legs and feet.

Other Office Ergonomic Practices I Use

My desk set-up is kind of weird, janky, and it's all pieced together. But I'm all about being FUNCTIONAL. In my own words, I define functional as "practical, rather than decorative, common, deferred, attractive, or 'normal'".

A functional ergonomic set-up is almost always unique for each person. It needs to be looked at on a case-by-case basis because there are many variables involved. For example, height of person, length of arms, length of legs, body composition, height of chair, depth of chair, and height of desk are just to name a few.

"Success is the sum of small efforts, repeated day in and day out."

-Robert Collier, 1885-1950
Author

My workstation is obsessive, yet highly underrated. Here are all the outside-the-box angles I take at ergonomics for a high speed, energetic work environment.

- A foam roller (to release muscle tension in the back from sitting all day)
- A lumbar support in my chair made of a mesh netting that conforms to different shapes/sizes
- A second lumbar support on top of that (because one support doesn't push me forward enough in my chair) which is an air pillow (also conforms to different shapes/sizes)
- A high speed, ergonomic keyboard tray I designed/constructed out of one simple piece of flat cardboard. I put my keyboard on top of the cardboard. It allows me to slide my keyboard closer to me, without falling off the desk. Your elbows should always be close to your sides, not pushed forward in front of your upper body. Overextending your arms forward will cause upper back pain in your scapulae. Also, overextending your elbows to the sides (just so they can rest on armrests) will cause repetitive strain injuries from the top of your neck all the way through your shoulder to your biceps and triceps.
- A foot rest that raises my feet slightly so that my legs and feet are at the correct angle. It also helps the leg muscles relax while I'm sitting.
- A 5 foot long (¾" diameter) PVC pipe for shoulder roll exercises to counteract upper back tension from constant internal shoulder rotation (from typing and using a mouse all day). A shoulder roll is when you (while standing straight up with good posture) hold the PVC pipe near your waist, with both hands and a wide grip. Then, you slowly raise

the pipe over your head with straight arms. Go all the way until the pipe touches your lower back or butt. Keep your arms straight at all times. Finally, do the opposite motion of what you just did to get the pipe back in the starting position. Then, repeat.

- A mini-fridge under my desk so I have no excuse not to prepare 4 to 5 small/medium sized meals/snacks per weekday.

Summary - Posture

Don't get discouraged if you try sitting with correct posture and it hurts or doesn't feel comfortable. It doesn't mean you aren't doing it right. It just means your body is being pulled out of bad habits (the way it's used to being held). It will get easier and easier as time goes on.

Start off taking small steps and making small improvements. The more muscle decompression you do (hot yoga, foam rolling, etc), the more comfortable you'll be when sitting with correct posture as time goes on. Remember, your muscles are tight from years, even hundreds and hundreds of hours of repetitive strain. It won't get fixed overnight. Be patient. It's the only option in my opinion. The only other alternative is to live a long life full of pain, while not using our body up to its full potential.

37

Breathing – Force Multiplier # 5

Welcome to the 5th and final part of my FORCE MULTIPLIER METHOD.

Reminder: this HIGH SPEED HEALTH FORCE MULTIPLIER METHOD was designed to inform athletes of how to change their everyday habits to prevent future repetitive stress injuries. Over time, these techniques will also make you an all-around healthier person, reducing stubborn mid-section body fat without even going to the gym. Each force multiplier you add to your equation of everyday habits increases your rate of success exponentially.

Incorporating these effective breathing strategies into your everyday habits will not be easy, but it's very attainable. Anything's possible, especially this, especially if you want to be successful badly enough. Stick with this technique and it will eventually become second nature. Once it does, the way you breathe will be one of the most effective force multipliers in building a strong balance between your abdomen and lower back. Eventually, it will instinctively promote good posture and reduce stubborn mid-section body fat. Since you breathe 24 hours a day, imagine strengthening your core and reducing fat from around your waist all day, with every breath you take, not just when you're in the gym. Here's how......

Old Misconception

There's an old misconception that your belly should expand when you take a deep breath. I used to practice this method for years. It was how I was taught. We were probably all taught that way. But, now I disagree with it. When your belly expands, it disengages your core muscles from supporting your body (putting unnecessary strain on your spine, back, neck, shoulders, hips, etc.).

When you take a deep breath, your lungs expand and fill up with air.

But take a look at where the lungs are located in the following image. You'll notice that the lungs are actually located inside the chest, not the belly. In fact, your lungs barely extend a little farther south below the bottom of your heart. Most people don't realize how high up their lungs really are in the chest.

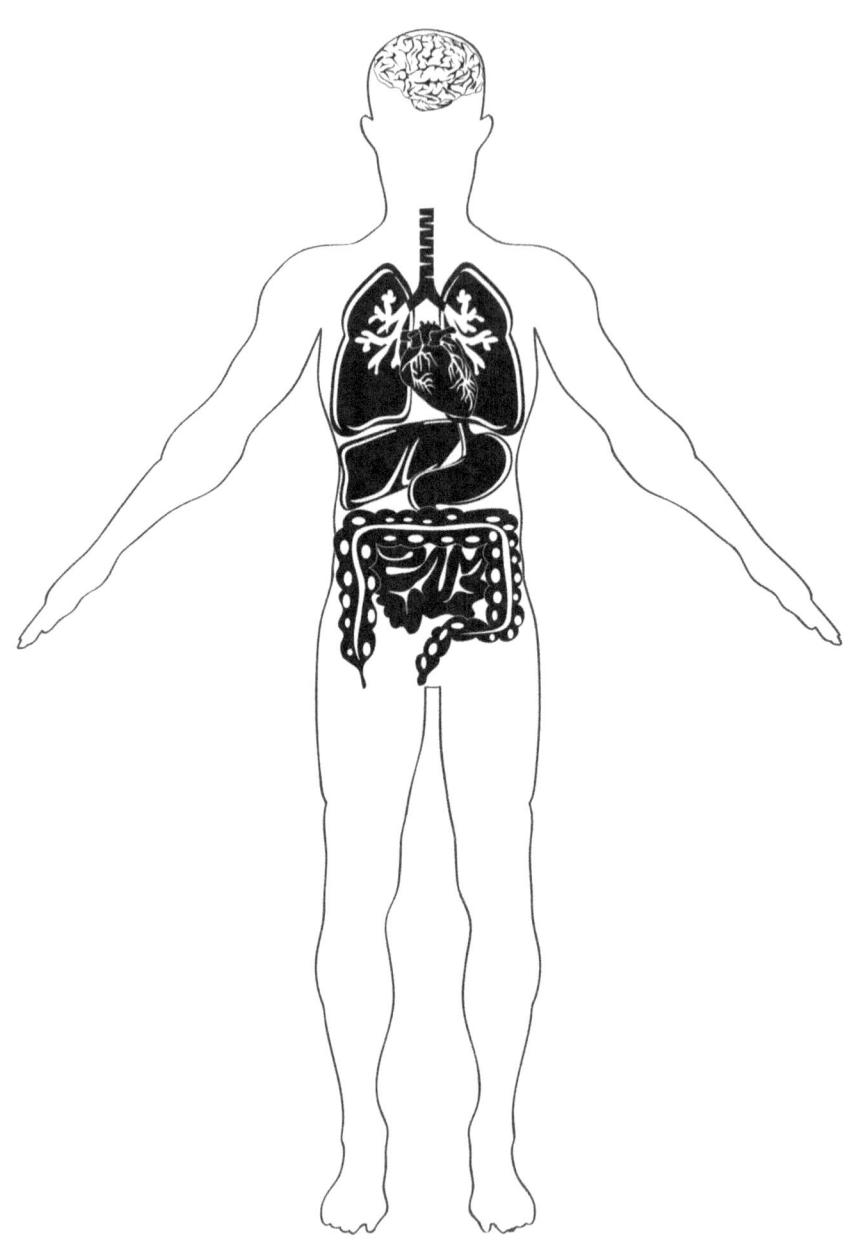

Now look at what's located inside your belly. Here you'll find the small intestine, large intestine, bladder, stomach, digestive system, etc. None of these body parts have any reason to expand when taking a deep breath. Your lungs, located inside your chest, are the only things taking in the air.

Therefore, focus on keeping your core engaged instead of letting your belly expand. At the same time, let your chest expand (instead of your belly) when you breathe in. Keep your core engaged both when breathing in and out. Imagine that you are pulling your belly button back toward your spine as hard as you can.

Practice Exercise

First things first, we must revisit the HSH FORCE MULTIPLIER METHOD's # 4 topic, Posture. This breathing technique is easiest to learn when standing.

- Stand up straight, knees relaxed and slightly bent.
- Leg muscles strong, supporting the majority of your body weight.
- Make sure your lower back has a slight lumbar curve in it.
- Scoop the bottom of your tailbone under towards the front of your body.
- Head should be directly over the rib cage (not leaned forward or back).
- Eyes looking directly ahead of you (not up or down to any degree), straight ahead.
- Shrug your shoulders straight up directly towards your ears.

- Then pull your shoulders straight back (behind you) as far as they'll go.
- Finally, pull your shoulders down toward the floor as far as they'll go, lock them in.
- You should feel the muscles in your mid-back contract right between your scapulae.

Now, you're ready to breathe correctly.

- Begin to breathe in deeply through your nose.
- While you breathe in, allow your chest and lungs to fill with air and expand.
- At the same time, keep your belly button pulled back in towards your spine as tight as you possibly can.
- When you're ready to exhale, breathe out through your mouth.
- While exhaling, let your chest return to the normal size it was before you started to inhale.
- Keep your core engaged and your belly button pulled in towards your spine the entire time.

If you're doing it correctly, you shouldn't be able to see your belly button at all (if you glance down). Your chest should be sticking out in front of your abdomen just far enough so that you can't see your belly button. If you CAN see your belly button, then you're standing with bad posture.

This technique can also be incorporated into your everyday routine when sitting, driving, exercising, sleeping, etc. It's just easiest to learn while standing up straight with correct posture.

Once this breathing technique becomes second nature to you, you'll notice significantly improved posture, more core strength, reduced pain/injury, and loss of that stubborn mid-section fat.

Section 4 -

Miscellaneous
Topics I'd Like to Cover

38

Sex (and It's Long-Term Physical Effects on the Body)

Ahhhhhh........sex. Such a beautiful thing. Especially when you work hard to feel great in your own skin, then you match up with a partner that's equally attractive and confident.

The few minutes after an orgasm are some of the most relaxing and satisfying moments a person can experience. Almost all of your muscles are relaxed and blood is circulating through parts of the body that blood flow is usually restricted.

But let's talk about the minutes leading up to that orgasm. It can take a lot of work for a person to reach climax. Most of the muscles used to complete that work are surrounding the sexual organs. As we all know, our sexual organs are located in our pelvis, and the main muscles in the front of the pelvis are the hips and core. The hips and core work overtime (10 minutes, 20 minutes, more....) when trying to reach climax. After climax, the rest of your body feels relaxed, but your hips and the lower portion of your abdomen are fried. They are so overworked, they don't even feel sore. It's more like a numb feeling. There's minimal blood flowing through these muscles because they've been overexerted past the point of muscle soreness. You don't even realize they are tight because they've been jacked up for so long that you're used to it by now. But, it's most likely causing pain in other areas of your body.

Now, take those same hip and lower ab muscles. Think about how much tension is created in them while you're sedentary, sitting at a desk all week long. These muscles are contracted for the majority of the week.

You go to the gym after work at night during the week and do some squats, but you don't stretch your hips out at all. Then, you get home on Friday night, have a few beers or alcoholic drinks to relax. That's right, you're dehydrated. Annnnd, now it's bed time. You hop in the sack with your mutually attractive partner and look forward to some good sex. You don't realize that you're about to tax your hip flexors past the point of being cooperative. You also don't realize that they've been contracted upwards of 40+ hours already, as well as hundreds of repetitions in the gym this week.

Hip muscles and the lower abdomen are probably the tightest muscles on the average athletic, sex-having desk jockey. They are compressed, pulling your groin muscle, quads, and IT bands. Your groin, quads, and IT bands are connected to tendons down at your knees. Exactly, if all these muscles are tight and inflexible, the only place to go is up. This pulls the tendons in the knees way too much. Now, Pes Anserine Tendonitis enters your life. Fun!

Everything I've mentioned in this section about sex has to do with muscles being compressed. Start using different decompression methods in these areas of muscle. Don't get discouraged when it takes a long time to get results (for muscles to start stretching and releasing). Keep in mind, you probably rarely ever stretch these muscles. Compare that to how many hours your hip muscles have been contracted in the last few years. It's going to be a long road to recovery, but you've got the rest of your life to do it. Get started now. Try not to get discouraged. The payoff is more than worth it.

39

The Smart Technology Craze and How It'll Lead to the Bad Neck Epidemic

There's no question about it, SMART Technology has changed my life for the better. For starters, I write my blog on my laptop and keep my iPad handy if I want to pull up an article, photo, video, email, notes, or search something on the Internet as I type on my computer. It pretty much doubles my productivity. Also, the ability to have (fast) Internet in our pocket, on a compact phone, was unimaginable 10 years ago.

But like the old saying goes, too much of a good thing can definitely be bad. Especially if you hold your iPad, iPhone, or other SMART device incorrectly when using it for long periods of time. Two major mistakes are (a) holding it in or near your lap when you're sitting straight up and (b) holding it on your chest when you're standing or lying flat on your back. Both of these mistakes cause your head to crank forward and your neck to be overextended (while looking too far down). It also causes a huge muscle imbalance in the neck. The muscles in the back of the neck are constantly stretched during these 2 common faults. Meanwhile, the muscles in the front of the neck are constantly contracted. Here's an analogy for all you weightlifters, it's like holding a bicep curl for an hour straight and never doing any tricep exercises.

Check out Exhibit A below. This guy's spinal cord has a normal/correct curvature to it. Check out how the spine inside his neck goes straight up into the air, then even angles back a slight degree, keeping the head properly balanced directly over the upper body.

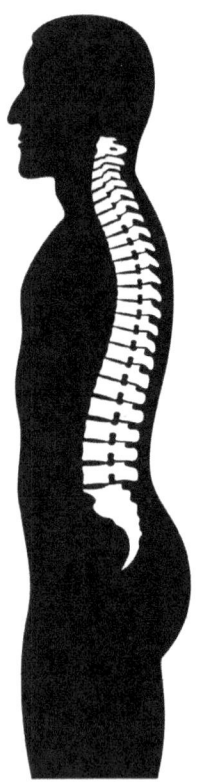

Now check out this unhappy camper, aka Exhibit B. Look at his neck and how his spine is permanently bowed forward. The spine in his neck is not even close to straight up in the air, let alone bowed backward slightly (like in Exhibit A). His head is in front of his upper body causing unnecessary tension and major neck pain. Finally, he'll never even know the damage he's done to his vertebrae and discs in his spine (neck area) until he gets an x-ray.

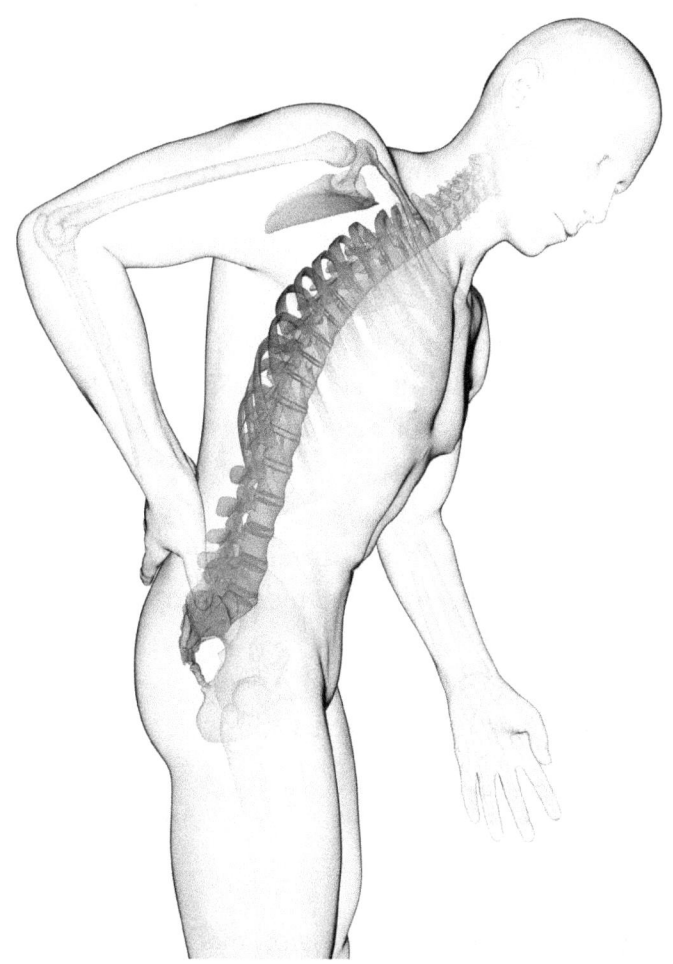

Don't think it's a big deal? Take my case for example. I knew I had tension issues in my neck, but I had no idea how serious it was or how dangerous of a path I started down. I also didn't have any neck pain. Until one day, I got rear-ended while sitting at a red light. It's OK, she was only driving a full-size Suburban and she only hit me twice since she was on her cell phone with her foot on the gas. Anyway, I feel a "How Not to Drive While Distracted" blog post coming up in the near future. Haha. Bottom line, the car accident led to me getting an x-ray and finding out that I was in the first stage of Spinal Degeneration in my neck (not related to the accident at all). There are 4 stages of Spinal Degeneration. It happens due to bad habits of repetitive strain over time, not a sudden accident or trauma. Spinal Degeneration is when the discs between the vertebrae start to erode away and the spine loses its natural curvature in the neck. I know, sounds fun.

Don't get me wrong, I obviously used to be a huge offender of these two postural flaws while using SMART technology. However, I've gotten a lot better at avoiding mistakes and overcompensating for them when possible.

In summary, there's nothing I can do to regenerate the discs in the back of my neck. But, what I can do to stop the progression of further spinal degeneration is:

1. Use correct posture as much as possible.

2. Avoid overextension of the neck for any significant period of time.

3. Practice multiple decompression methods to make sure the muscles in my neck are proportionately balanced.

40

The Physical Effects of Mental and Emotional Stress

I'd like to thank y'all for making it through some of the wacky analogies I've given you so far in this book. That said, here is the final (and possibly the weirdest) one.

Picture this, if you've done sit-ups or crunches in your life, you know how physically taxing they can be. But have you ever held that sit-up, or crunch, in the contracted position for a few seconds to get the extra burn and extra results? Or have you ever done a plank and held it for a while (upwards of a minute)? If so, you'll be able to relate to this one.

You wake up on a weekday from a somewhat comfortable, relaxing night of sleep. You don't want to get out of bed, even though you're wide awake, because you're thinking about the stress you have ahead of you in your work day. Your brain is already working a mile a minute, whether you're being productive or not. The first major muscle group leading away from your brain is your neck. Depending on your position, either the front, back, or sides of your neck are extremely contracted and going through loads of unnecessary muscle tension. These muscles are directly connected to the muscles in your shoulders and upper back, contracting all of them as well. Then, you drive to work crouched up tightly in your car, mad about every stoplight you catch and every knucklehead out there pulling stunts and cutting you off. Finally, you make it to work. The thought of sitting at your desk makes you want to cringe. You guessed it. Your neck and shoulders are still contracted due to this mental stress and they're going to stay that way for the majority of the next 8 to 9 hours. This mental stress is taking a huge toll on your body physically.

You have no idea about this over-tension because you're so used to it and you can't even feel it. However, you could feel the burn in your abdomen a couple days ago when you were holding that crunch tight or holding that minute long plank. Why could you feel the burn in your abs, but not feel the burn in your neck, shoulders, and upper back in this situation? Your abs are rarely ever in that contracted position for that long, but your neck and shoulders are in that position very often. You don't realize the effects of how bad it is because it's past the point of inefficiency.

The same goes for emotional stress. Intimate relationships, strained friendships, the death of a loved one....all of these are examples of emotional stress that takes a physical toll on the body. They start in the head, tension goes directly to the neck, then the shoulders, and then it travels throughout your whole body. As I said earlier in this book, every muscle in your body is connected in one way or another. Everything. A tight right shoulder could be the cause of a pain in your neck. A tight muscle in the left side of your back could be the cause of a pain in your right knee. I can't tell you how many times I've foam rolled my neck and it caused my lower back or one of my hips to pop into place.

I know, this all sounds crazy but it's true. There are hundreds, even thousands, of possibilities of what could be the source and what could be the end result of pain. Mental and emotional stresses cause unhealthy muscle compression just as much, if not more, than physical activity.

41

The Power and Ability of Human Healing - Closing Thoughts

The human body is an incredibly fascinating system. You would think that we'd be able to appreciate it by simply living inside it every day for 30-some years. However, there's so much out there for us to learn. In my opinion, the keys to success are longevity, creativity, and repetition. All three of these factors are crucial.

Longevity - Make permanent lifestyle changes for the better as opposed to temporary fixes.

Creativity - Change it up. Think outside-the-box. If something isn't working, try something completely different. Don't do more and more of something that isn't working for you.

Repetition - Find what works and make sure you enjoy it. Success is much more attainable when you're doing something you enjoy and are passionate about. Do this over and over. And over. And over. And over.

By investing time and taking full responsibility for our own bodies, our quality of life and physique will skyrocket. Never stop learning. The day you stop learning, the results are all downhill from there. Do something every single day that will get you closer to your goal. Regardless of how big or small the task, take at least one step forward every single day. We've been subjected to years and years of repetitive strain. In order to even start counteracting that, we need to be passionate and powerful about holistic healing. The healing capability of the human body is far more advanced than any of us can ever imagine.

You could've done anything in the world just now, but you took the time to read my book. For that, I'm very grateful and would like to thank you. I hope it's showed you the importance of taking a well-rounded, holistic approach to your future health and wellness.

You only live once. Do what you love, take care, and stay functional.

Life's good and anything's possible. Anything.

Todd Bowen
www.highspeedhealth.com

HIGH SPEED HEALTH
A Quick and Direct Guide to Healing Pain
Caused by Repetitive Strain Injuries
For the Part-Time Athlete
Who Sits at a Desk Full-Time

Free Report

The book is over, but the content never stops.

Go download my free running report at www.highspeedhealth.com/freereport.

It's only available to readers who've purchased my book.

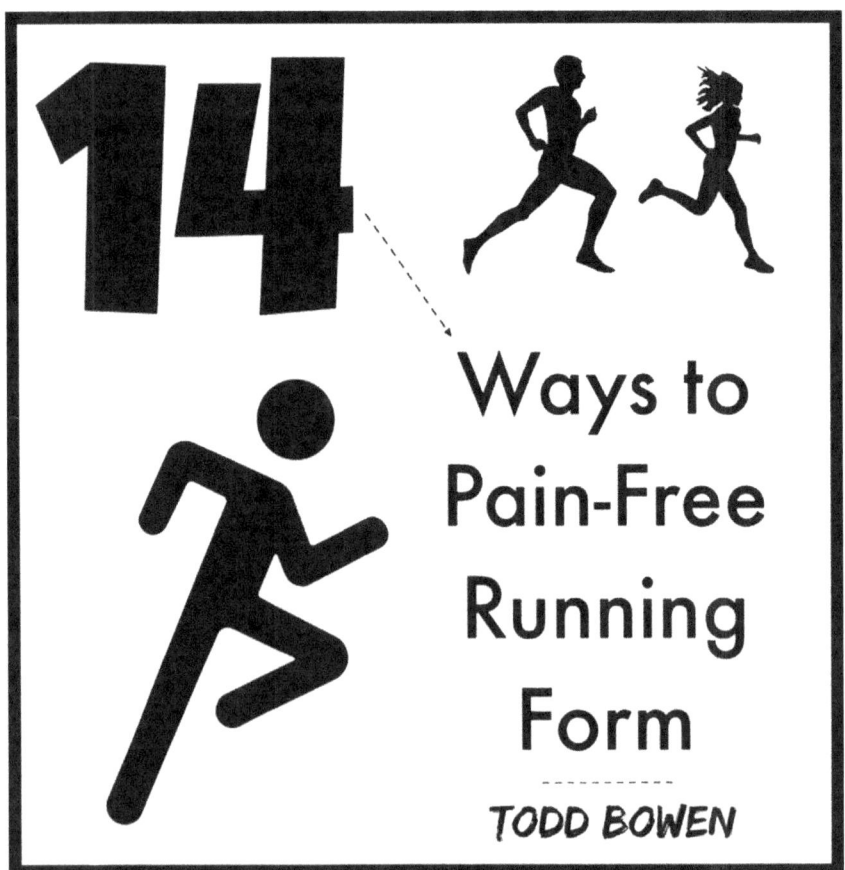

Improve your running form at www.highspeedhealth.com/freereport.

www.ingramcontent.com/pod-product-compliance
Lightning Source LLC
Chambersburg PA
CBHW070144290526
45789CB00002B/621